CONTRACEPTION
AND
REPRODUCTION

Health Consequences
for Women and Children
in the Developing World

Working Group on the Health Consequences of
Contraceptive Use and Controlled Fertility

Committee on Population
Commission on Behavioral and Social Sciences and Education
National Research Council

NATIONAL ACADEMY PRESS
Washington, D.C. 1989

NATIONAL ACADEMY PRESS • 2101 Constitution Avenue, NW • Washington, DC 20418

Library of Congress Catalog Card No. 89-63004
International Standard Book Number 0-309-04094-9

Additional copies of this report are available from:

National Academy Press
2101 Constitution Avenue, NW
Washington, DC 20418

Printed in the United States of America
S028

Working Group on the Health Consequences of Contraceptive Use and Controlled Fertility

WILLIAM FOEGE (*Chair*), Carter Presidential Center, Atlanta, Ga.
JULIE DaVANZO (*Cochair*), Economics and Statistics Department, The RAND Corporation, Santa Monica, Calif.
JOHN BONGAARTS, The Population Council, New York
RONALD GRAY, Department of Population Dynamics, Johns Hopkins University
JOHN E. KNODEL, Population Studies Center, University of Michigan
JORGE MARTINEZ-MANAUTOU, Family Planning Services, Mexican Institute of Social Security
ANNE R. PEBLEY, Office of Population Research, Princeton University
ALLAN G. ROSENFIELD, School of Public Health, Columbia University
BRUCE V. STADEL, Epidemiology Branch, Food and Drug Administration, Rockville, Md.

PETER J. DONALDSON, Study Director
ALLAN M. PARNELL, Research Associate
SUSAN M. ROGERS, Research Associate
DIANE L. GOLDMAN, Administrative Assistant

iii

Committee on Population

Preface

This report is one of a series of studies that have been carried out under the auspices of the Committee on Population to examine the consequences of changes in demographic behavior, particularly as they influence the lives of people in the developing world. In 1986 a working group of the committee released a landmark study of the consequences of population growth for the economic development of the Third World. This report concentrates on what many analysts regard as an equally important aspect of the demographic behavior of couples in developing countries, namely, the health consequences of different patterns of childbearing and contraceptive use.

This report focuses on the health effects for mothers and their children of changes in the timing of pregnancies, the interval between them, and the number of children women have. In addition, it provides an overview of what is known about the health risks and benefits of different contraceptive methods used in the developing world. Throughout, the report focuses on the consequences that changes in the number and spacing of pregnancies and the ages of childbearing would have on the health of individual women and children, their families, and the larger population. This report and the research on which it is based deal almost entirely with the situation in the developing world, in countries that are characterized by low per capita income and limited health services.

On the basis of a comprehensive review of the available evidence, the working group concludes that reproductive patterns exercise an important influence on the health of women and children. Moreover, the working group believes that a series of public policy measures related to reproduction could be undertaken that would improve the health of mothers and children in developing countries. In the view of the working group, improving the performance of family planning programs may have significant effects on the health of women and children.

We have written this report for a scientific audience. It will probably be most congenial and most useful to researchers actively involved in studies of the relationship between reproduction and health in developing countries. In addition, we hope that the report will be useful to others: to policy makers who may be concerned about the possible utility of family planning programs as a health intervention, as well as to students, both in the United States and throughout the developing world, who are interested in the relationship between health and reproduction, whether they are in research-oriented programs or in training in public health or clinical service. Although the report is undeniably technical in orientation and approach, we have attempted, through the executive summary, the glossary, and the style of presentation throughout, to make it accessible to a wide audience.

In carrying out its study, the working group commissioned experts in the field to prepare background papers. These papers, which are listed in the appendix, deal with specific topics related to health and fertility, and they contributed significantly to this report. A volume containing the papers of greatest interest will be published separately later this year.

The committee and the working group very much appreciate the efforts of those who prepared these background papers. The paper by Susan Zimicki provided a basis for Chapter 3. The paper by Nancy Lee, Herbert Peterson, and Susan Cho provided a basis for Chapter 4. The paper by John Haaga provided the basis for parts of Chapter 5. Chapter 6 is an expanded version of a draft initially prepared by James McCarthy. The other background papers were also influential in the working group's deliberations and in the drafting of this report.

The Working Group on Health Consequences of Contraceptive Use and Controlled Fertility met six times to discuss the background papers, to review the relevant scientific literature and other studies of similar topics that were under way or recently completed, and to discuss and review the various drafts of this report. In addition, working group member Anne Pebley spent much of the summer of 1988 working full-time on this report at the Committee on Population's offices. Each member of the working group also participated in several smaller, less formal meetings during which specific aspects of the report were reviewed.

The Committee on Population undertook this study at the request of the Agency for International Development (AID), which asked for an authoritative assessment of the health consequences of the changing patterns of fertility and the increasing use of modern contraceptives that have been taking place in developing countries as an aid in designing its program of assistance to developing countries. The Rockefeller Foundation also provided significant support for this project through a grant to the Committee on Population; the Rockefeller Foundation support allowed considerable flexibility in preparing the report and facilitated wide dissemination by making possible translations of the report into Spanish and French. The William and Flora Hewlett Foundation also provided support for the working group through a grant to the Committee on Population.

The committee and the working group appreciate the work provided by Peter J. Donaldson, study director, and Susan M. Rogers, research associate. Special thanks are also due Allan McMillan Parnell, research associate, who had principal responsibility for coordinating the preparation of this report. Laurence Grummer-Strawn, who served as a research assistant to the working group during the summer of 1988, also made important contributions to the report. Jeremiah Sullivan and Ann Way, of the Demographic and Health Surveys, provided some of the data used in Chapter 6. Michael Koenig provided data on infant and maternal mortality from Bangladesh. Carol Bradford skillfully prepared all figures in the report. Sivaporn Pokpong, a student at the University of Michigan, Audrey Vanden Heuvel, a student at the University of North Carolina, Irma Elo, a student at Princeton University, and Lisa Brecker all assisted in compilation of materials and preparation of tables. The committee and the working group especially appreciate the help received from Christine L. McShane, editor of the Commission on Behavioral and Social Sciences and Education.

The working group responsible for this report was composed of a carefully selected, balanced group of experts with backgrounds in both medical and social sciences. The Committee on Population is very grateful to the members of this group for their hard work, and particularly to William Foege and Julie DaVanzo, who served as chair and cochair, respectively, and to Anne Pebley, whose concentrated effort contributed greatly to the report.

ALBERT I. HERMALIN, *Chair*
Committee on Population

Contents

Executive Summary

Family planning programs have been developed and supported to provide people with a means to achieve the number of children they desire and to reduce unwanted pregnancy, as a means of improving the health of women and children, and to contribute to slower population growth and more rapid economic development. In 1987 the National Research Council's Committee on Population appointed the Working Group on the Health Consequences of Contraceptive Use and Controlled Fertility to assess what is known about the health risks and benefits of contraceptive methods, about the effects of reproductive patterns (numbers, timing, and spacing of births) on women's and children's health, and about the likely effects on the health of women and children of trends and differences in reproductive patterns in the developing world.

The working group concluded that family planning programs contribute to the improvement of the health of women and children in developing countries by providing safe and effective means for women to reduce the number of births and high-risk pregnancies they have. Family planning may also improve the health of infants by increasing the spacing between births. Easy access to family planning services and improved provision of these services should be encouraged, particularly in conjunction with efforts to increase access to prenatal care, to encourage breastfeeding, and to advance other health services. In countries in which safe abortion is not available, family planning services are even more important from a health standpoint because they provide a medically sound way to reduce unwanted pregnancies that could otherwise lead to maternal death or injury from dangerous abortion procedures.

1

REPRODUCTIVE PATTERNS AND MATERNAL HEALTH

Research conducted in developing countries demonstrates that maternal age and parity are associated with maternal health. In particular, maternal mortality may be reduced by:

- Reducing the total number of pregnancies each woman has;
- Reducing the number of high-parity births;
- Reducing the number of births to very young and older women;
- Reducing the use of abortion to terminate unwanted pregnancies in countries in which safe abortion is unavailable; and
- Reducing the number of pregnancies to women with major health problems.

CONTRACEPTIVE RISKS AND BENEFITS

Modern contraceptives are an important means through which women in developing countries control their fertility. On the basis of our review of the scientific evidence concerning the risks and benefits of contraception, we conclude that the risks associated with the use of currently available modern contraceptive methods are considerably lower than the risks associated with pregnancy, labor and delivery, particularly in developing countries. Moreover, research has increasingly demonstrated direct health benefits of contraceptive use. Although these results are based largely on studies conducted in the developed world, we regard the available research as a reasonable guide to the risks and benefits of contraceptive use in the developing world.

REPRODUCTIVE PATTERNS AND CHILDREN'S HEALTH

A large and growing number of studies in the developing world demonstrate that the spacing between births, maternal age, and birth order are associated with child health and survival. In some cases the causal mechanisms influencing these relationships are not fully understood. Nevertheless, the weight of evidence suggests that infant and child mortality may be reduced by:

- Reducing the number of births that occur within approximately two years of a previous birth;
- Reducing the number of children born to very young mothers;
- Reducing the number of children born to women in poor health; and
- Reducing the number of higher-order births.

Children born following unwanted pregnancies may also be at increased health risk, but the evidence is incomplete.

HEALTH CONSEQUENCES OF CHANGING REPRODUCTIVE PATTERNS FOR COUNTRIES

Declining fertility will improve the health of women in a society by reducing the number of pregnancies and births and therefore the exposure to risk. Other changes in reproductive patterns will improve the health of women and children to the degree that high-risk pregnancies and births are reduced. Some of the changes that are likely to take place will reduce certain high-risk births while at the same time increasing others. For example, as a society's level of fertility drops, the proportion of high-risk, higher-order births will decrease, but the proportion of high-risk first births will increase. The effect of an increase in the proportion of high-risk first births can be mitigated by an increase in the age at which women begin childbearing, especially in societies where a large proportion of women have their first birth at very young ages.

Whether spacing between births will widen or narrow as fertility declines is not clear; both patterns are found in the few countries for which data for more than one point in time are available. Changes in fertility may be associated with an increase in the proportion of short birth intervals if declines in breastfeeding are not offset by increased contraceptive use. Although more research on the relationship between contraceptive use and breastfeeding is needed, programs designed to encourage both breastfeeding and contraceptive use for birth spacing are likely to have important health benefits for children.

1

Introduction

This report examines the scientific evidence regarding the consequences of reproductive patterns for the health of women and children in developing countries. Reproductive patterns refer to the ages at which women give birth, the lengths of time between births, and the total number of births a woman has. Because reproductive patterns in developing countries have been influenced greatly by use of modern contraceptives, the risks and benefits of different contraceptive methods are also evaluated. Although some of the data on which our analysis is based have been drawn from research in developed countries, the focus of the report is the developing world.

The chapters that follow address three fundamental questions:

1. What are the relationships between contraceptive use and reproductive patterns, on one hand, and women's and children's health, on the other?

2. What have been the effects of differences and changes in reproductive patterns on differentials and changes in women's and children's health?

3. What is the potential for family planning to bring about (further) improvements in women's and children's health?

Answers to these three questions have important implications for health and family planning programs throughout the developing world because they help determine appropriate levels of resources to allocate to these programs. Questions about the relationships among fertility, contraceptive use, and health are also of considerable interest to population scientists, independent of their policy implications. The relationship between fertility and mortality is a fundamental aspect of the transition from a pattern of high mortality and high fertility charac-

5

teristic of traditional agrarian societies to the pattern of low mortality and low fertility found in contemporary industrial societies. This report examines how the health of women and children changes as a society moves from a situation in which no effort is made to control fertility to one in which women are concerned about the number and spacing of their pregnancies and use modern contraceptives to regulate both. It is during this transition that some of the most important health effects of changing fertility may be found.

THE DEMOGRAPHIC CONTEXT

This report examines aspects of the remarkable demographic changes that have occurred throughout the developing world over the last several decades. Mortality in developing countries, particularly among infants and children, is substantially lower today than it was three decades ago. Major declines in fertility have also taken place in many, although by no means all, developing countries. Increased availability and use of modern contraceptives and later ages at marriage and first birth are among the most important factors in contributing to these fertility declines. But, despite the declines in fertility and mortality that have occurred, large differences in the levels of fertility and mortality remain between the developing and the more developed world.

On average, women in developing countries have more than twice as many children as women in developed countries. The average life expectancy at birth (see the glossary for a definition) in the developing world is 14 years less than life expectancy at birth in developed countries. During the first half of the 1980s, the average rate of infant mortality in the developing world was almost six times the level found in the more developed countries. More than 13 percent of the children born in the developing world die before age 5, compared with less than 2 percent of the children in more developed countries. About 15 million children, 98 percent of them in developing countries, are estimated to have died each year from 1980 to 1985 (United Nations, 1988b).

Precise data on maternal mortality, that is, on deaths during pregnancy and childbirth, are more difficult to obtain, but it is clear that maternal mortality is also much higher in developing than in developed countries. Figure 1.1 is a map of maternal mortality around the world. It shows that a woman's lifetime risk of maternal death ranges from greater than 1 in 25 in parts of Africa to considerably less than 1 in 1,000 in the United States, Canada, and Western and Northern Europe.

Despite the trend toward overall lower mortality and fertility in developing countries, there is a substantial diversity in levels of mortality and fertility. Trends in infant mortality from 1955 through 1985 by geographic region are shown in Figure 1.2, and trends in child mortality (that is, deaths before age 5) are shown in Figure 1.3. According to the United Nations (1988b), the average probability of dying before age 1 declined by over 50 percent during this period in

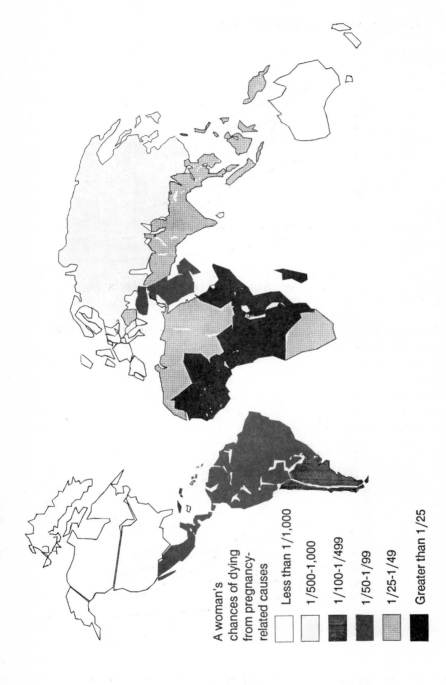

A woman's
chances of dying
from pregnancy-
related causes

☐ Less than 1/1,000

☐ 1/500-1,000

☐ 1/100-1/499

☐ 1/50-1/99

☐ 1/25-1/49

☐ Greater than 1/25

FIGURE 1.1 A woman's lifetime risk of maternal death, by region. Source: C. Lettenmaier et al. (1988).

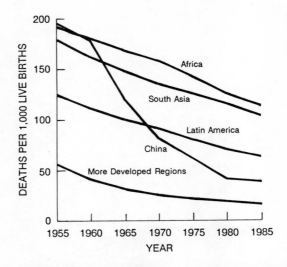

FIGURE 1.2   Infant mortality rates, by region, 1955-1985. Source: United Nations (1988b: Table A.2, pp. 36-41).

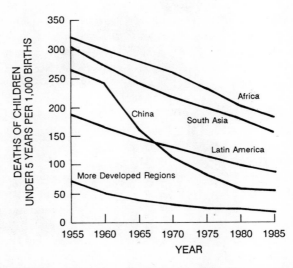

FIGURE 1.3   Child mortality rates, by region, 1955-1985. Source: United Nations (1988b: Table A.1, pp. 30-33).

less developed countries, with declines ranging from 29 percent in Eastern Africa to 80 percent in China. The average probability of dying before age 5 in less developed regions decreased by 52 percent, with Eastern Africa (29 percent) and China (79 percent) again being the regions of least and greatest improvement. Although comparable data are not available, maternal mortality also appears to have decreased substantially during the last three decades in some regions. Sivard (1985) estimates that maternal mortality in Latin America declined by almost half from 1960 to 1978. However, maternal mortality has remained high in Africa and South Asia.

With the exception of sub-Saharan Africa, fertility declined in every region during the last two decades. Concomitantly, contraceptive use has increased significantly in areas experiencing declines in fertility. Figure 1.4 shows that substantial increases in contraceptive prevalence occurred both in countries where initial levels of use were high and in countries where use was low. The increase in contraceptive use has been rapid in some countries, such as Thailand, but much slower in others, such as Egypt and Pakistan.

FAMILY PLANNING IN DEVELOPING COUNTRIES

The increase in contraceptive use in developing countries is due in part to government support for family planning services, which has increased the availability of contraceptives. In the early days of organized family planning in the developing world, the primary rationale for such support was that increasing contraceptive use would lower fertility, thereby slowing rapid population growth, which in turn would facilitate economic and social development. Government planners, policy makers, and many politicians accepted the argument that slowing aggregate rates of population growth would accelerate economic development. Public support has also been provided because the ability to determine the number and spacing of one's children has been increasingly recognized as a basic human right.

In addition to promoting contraceptive use for development and human rights reasons, many governments have also encouraged family planning as a means of improving the health of women and children. Health issues have long been the major concern in some areas, notably throughout Latin America. Over the years the health benefits of increased contraceptive use and lower fertility have become the most important policy objectives for a number of developing countries and for many of the international agencies that support family planning programs. This increased interest in the health consequences of changing fertility has been encouraged both by a growing awareness of the potential benefits that lower fertility and better spacing of pregnancies may have on maternal and child health and by an increasing eagerness by politicians to work to improve health. While the number and timing of pregnancies have long been regarded as factors affecting women's health, it was not until the early 1970s that a significant number of

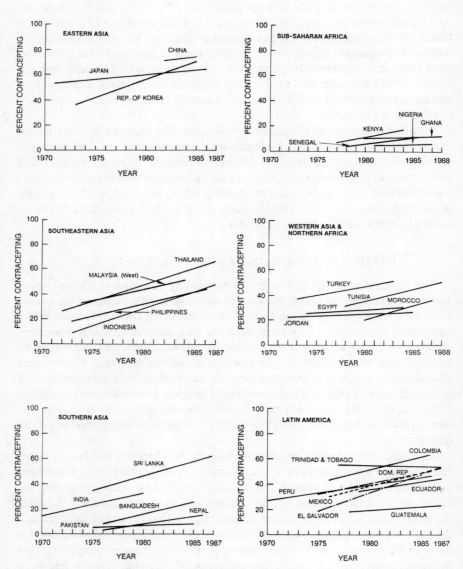

FIGURE 1.4   Contraceptive prevalence trends (percentage of married women ages 15-49 currently using contraceptive methods), 1970-1987.   Source: United Nations (1988a).

studies began to examine the relationship between different patterns of fertility and women's and children's health.

The advances in contraceptive technology, in particular the widespread use of the birth control pill and the intrauterine device (IUD), that contributed to the diffusion of family planning also raised questions about the health effects associated with prolonged use of some methods. The real and perceived health risks of different contraceptives are cited by some health professionals in developing countries as reasons to place restrictions on certain contraceptives, as well as by some couples in developing countries as their reason for being reluctant to control their fertility using modern contraceptives. Contraceptive methods have continued to evolve as efforts are made to reduce health risks and improve efficacy, and research increasingly has demonstrated direct health benefits associated with the use of some contraceptive methods.

ORGANIZATION OF THE REPORT

Given the widespread changes that have taken place, it is important for both scientific and policy reasons to assess the scientific evidence available on the relationships among contraceptive use, reproductive patterns, and health.

The remainder of the report is organized as follows. Chapter 2 provides an overview of the hypothesized relationships between reproductive patterns and the health of women and children. Chapter 3 examines the evidence on the effects of pregnancy and reproductive patterns on women's health and survival. Chapter 4 assesses the health risks and benefits of different contraceptive methods that may be used to control fertility. Chapter 5 evaluates the evidence on the effects of different reproductive patterns on children's health and survival. Chapter 6 describes the changes in reproductive patterns that have taken place across the developing world. Chapter 7 presents the implications of the working group's analysis for family planning policy and for future research. A glossary of technical terms related to reproduction and contraception completes the report.

2

Hypotheses About Reproductive Patterns and Women's and Children's Health

In developing countries, where resources are scarce, health services are poor and not readily available, and infectious diseases are common, it is difficult to maintain good health. Although the primary causes of poor health in such an environment are often beyond the control of individual families (at least in the short run), there are ways in which they can act to reduce the risk of illness and death. Choosing to limit fertility, to delay the onset of childbearing, to space births, and to breastfeed are among the actions that may reduce the risk of illness and death to women and children.

The central objective of this report is to assess the effects of particular reproductive patterns for the health of women and children. Of course, reproductive patterns are not a direct cause of death, in the way hemorrhage or infectious diseases are, but rather they may be associated with conditions leading to death. The chapter begins by examining hypotheses about the direct effects of reproductive patterns, first on women's health, then on children's health. By direct effects we mean the biological and behavioral mechanisms through which a change in childbearing patterns might affect women's and children's health directly. Next, we discuss hypothesized indirect effects of changes in reproduction on women and children's health. Indirect effects refer to changes in household structure and parental roles and new or foregone opportunities that are a consequence of changes in the number and timing of births that may themselves influence health.

While the report focuses primarily on possible direct and indirect effects of reproductive patterns on women's and children's health, interaction or synergistic effects may also be operating. In these cases, the presence of two conditions or behaviors alters their effects. For example, the joint detrimental consequences of

12

using oral contraceptives and smoking are noted in Chapter 4. Numerous other interaction effects may be occurring, but they are beyond the scope of this report.

We then review other possible explanations for relationships between reproductive patterns and health, such as the possibility that other health behaviors (e.g., use of modern medical care) affect both reproductive patterns and health. Finally, we discuss the types of evidence on which our findings are based.

DIRECT EFFECTS OF REPRODUCTIVE PATTERNS ON HEALTH

Reproductive Patterns and Women's Health

Practicing physicians and midwives have observed that women who have many children and women with certain reproductive patterns are at higher risk of poor health and mortality. These observed relationships may be directly causal or may be due to confounding factors. In addition, it is possible that the poorer health of certain women or their children may lead to certain reproductive patterns, such as reduced fertility. Hypotheses concerning the effects of reproductive patterns on the health of women are summarized in Table 2.1.

There are at least five reasons to believe that women who limit their fertility will have better health. First, each time a woman becomes pregnant, she is at risk of pregnancy complications and related complications that she does not face when she is not pregnant. Thus, over the course of a lifetime, women who have many children are more likely than women who have fewer children to experience reproductive illness or mortality—merely because they are exposed more often to the risks associated with each pregnancy. The risks associated with pregnancy include pregnancy-induced hypertension, ectopic pregnancy, hemorrhage, obstructed labor, infection, and, for those not wanting to be pregnant, the hazards of unsafe abortion. The health benefits of fewer pregnancies are likely to be greater in regions where prenatal and intrapartum care are poor, because the risks associated with each pregnancy are greater. These issues are discussed in greater detail in Chapter 3.

Second, in addition to having fewer pregnancies, women who control their fertility can avoid pregnancies that may pose higher-than-normal risks to their health. Research suggests that women who have had many previous pregnancies may be at higher risk of poor health from a given pregnancy than women who are pregnant for the second, third, or fourth time. Women who have had many previous pregnancies may be at higher risk of morbidity and mortality because of the cumulative toll of previous pregnancies and because of previous reproductive injury. In particular, they may be more likely to experience complications such as uterine rupture and hemorrhage than women who have had fewer previous pregnancies.

The first pregnancy also appears to have a higher risk than the second, third, or fourth pregnancy. Women who are having their first child appear to be at higher

TABLE 2.1 Hypothesized Direct Effects of Reproductive Patterns on Women's Health

Reproductive Pattern	Hypothesized Effect
Number of pregnancies	Each pregnancy carries a risk of reproductive morbidity and mortality
High-risk pregnancies	
First pregnancies	Adaptation to pregnancy for the first time
High-order pregnancies	Hemorrhage; uterine rupture; previous reproductive injury
Pregnancy at very young maternal ages	Inadequate development of reproductive system and incomplete growth
	Adequate prenatal and interpartum care less likely
Pregnancy at older ages	Body in poorer condition for pregnancy and childbirth
Short interbirth intervals	Inadequate time to rebuild nutritional stores and regain energy level
Unwanted pregnancies ending in unsafe abortion	Abortions performed by unsafe means increase exposure to injury, infection, hemorrhage, and death
Large family size	Reduced availability of family resources for women's health and nutrition
Pregnancies for women already in poor health	Aggravated health condition
Use of contraception	Direct health risks and benefits associated with contraceptive methods

risk of obstructed labor, pregnancy-induced hypertension, and birth complications. However, since any woman who has children must have a first birth, women who desire children obviously cannot choose to avoid first pregnancies in order to lower their risks of morbidity or mortality.

Reproductive morbidity and mortality may also be more common for women who become pregnant at the very beginning and at the end of their reproductive years. Pregnancy may be more stressful physiologically to very young women, because their reproductive systems are not yet fully mature and they may not yet have completed their growth. Young girls may also be less likely to detect a pregnancy early on or, for a variety of reasons, they may deny the pregnancy. In both cases they may seek prenatal care later in pregnancy than desirable or delay having an abortion (in situations where either is available). Older women may encounter problems more frequently during pregnancy and birth because the ability of their reproductive systems to cope with the burden of pregnancy has declined with age. Evidence of decline in the function of the reproductive system with maternal age includes an increased incidence of fetal chromosomal abnormalities and spontaneous abortion.

Pregnancies that begin shortly after a previous birth may also pose higher risks for women. Short interbirth intervals, especially if accompanied by intensive breastfeeding, may prevent a woman from rebuilding depleted nutritional stores before the next pregnancy begins. This problem is likely to be more serious among women who are malnourished to begin with and may be exacerbated by a sequence of closely spaced pregnancies.

A pregnancy that occurs when a woman's health is already jeopardized is likely to pose a greater risk than a pregnancy for a healthy woman. Women who are malnourished, who are seriously ill, or who have chronic health conditions are clearly at higher risk than healthier women. By avoiding pregnancy, women with health problems may substantially improve their own chances for survival and good health.

Third, in addition to reducing the total number of pregnancies and avoiding potentially higher-risk pregnancies, women in many developing countries can also substantially reduce their risk of reproductive morbidity and mortality by using contraception to avoid unwanted pregnancies rather than resort to unsafe abortion to terminate such pregnancies. In many developing countries, abortion is illegal and is often performed by untrained personnel in unhygienic conditions. Abortions attempted by women themselves or performed by abortionists under septic conditions substantially increase a woman's risk of infection, injury or hemorrhage, and death.

The three hypothesized mechanisms just described suggest that changes in reproductive patterns may improve health by decreasing exposure to infection, injury, and other reproductive complications. A fourth possible mechanism is the use of contraception itself, which may affect women's health. There may also be a fifth and more general effect of changes in reproductive patterns on women's health. Most families in developing countries have limited resources that must be allocated to a variety of family needs. Families with fewer young children to care for are likely to have more resources (including time, food, and money) to devote to the health of each family member. For example, women in smaller families may have more time to go to a clinic for treatment of an illness or for a prenatal visit.

Reproductive Patterns and Children's Health

A woman's reproductive pattern may also have important effects on the health and survival chances of her children. Children's well-being, especially in the first year of life, is highly dependent on their mothers' health during and after pregnancy. For this reason, some of the hypothesized effects of reproductive patterns on children's health are closely related to the effects of reproductive patterns on women's health. Specifically, children who are firstborn or are of high birth order, children born into larger families, children born to very young or older mothers, children born after short previous interbirth intervals or before a short subsequent interbirth interval, and children who were unwanted at the time they were conceived may be at higher risk of poor health and mortality than other children. It is also possible that a mother's use of contraception may affect her child's health directly, for example through effects on lactation. These hypotheses are summarized in Table 2.2.

Birth Order

Since nulliparous women experience more problems during pregnancy, first-born children may be less healthy at birth, may weigh less at birth (because of poorer intrauterine growth or shorter gestation), and may experience more trauma during birth. The parents of firstborn children may also be less experienced in child care, although this explanation for poorer health among firstborns seems less plausible in societies in which new parents frequently live with older, more experienced relatives. Reducing the number of first births that women have is obviously not a sensible policy objective, since families choosing to have children must have a first birth, but delaying first births could be an important policy objective, particularly for very young women.

Children born of higher-order pregnancies may experience higher risks of morbidity and mortality for at least two reasons. First, as discussed above, because of the cumulative toll of numerous previous pregnancies and associated breastfeeding on maternal nutritional stores (described as the "maternal depletion syndrome"), mothers of higher-order children may be in poorer health prior to and during pregnancy, as well as after birth. Women who have reached high parity (fifth and higher parity) are also more likely to have experienced injuries during childbirth, which may complicate a higher-order pregnancy and birth. Thus, higher-order children may be at greater risk of poor intrauterine growth, greater trauma during birth, and, more generally, poorer health than children born at orders 2, 3, and 4. Second, children born at higher orders may be in poorer health because their families have fixed resources (such as time, money, food, and shelter) and more children to care for with these resources. On one hand, the sixth or seventh child in a poor family may receive less time and attention from parents than the first or second child did at a comparable age because there are now many children who need attention. On the other hand, older children may help to care

TABLE 2.2 Hypothesized Direct Effects of Reproductive Patterns on Children's Health

Reproductive Pattern	Hypothesized Effect
Firstborn children	More frequent maternal problems during pregnancy and childbirth; parents have less experience with child care; poorer intrauterine growth
Higher-order children	Maternal depletion; cumulative effect of earlier maternal reproductive injury; poorer intrauterine growth
Large families	Limited family resources allocated to more children; spread of infection among family members
Children born to very young mothers	Inadequate development of maternal reproductive system and incomplete maternal growth; young mothers less likely to receive adequate prenatal and intrapartum care or to provide good child care
Children born to older mothers	Greater risk of birth trauma; greater risk of genetic abnormalities
Short interbirth intervals	Inadequate maternal recovery time (maternal depletion); competition among similar aged siblings for limited family resources; early termination of breastfeeding; low birthweight; increased exposure to infection from children of similar ages
Unwantedness	(Conscious or unconscious) neglect; child born into a stressful situation
Maternal death or illness (e.g., chronic infection such as AIDS)	Early termination of breastfeeding; no maternal care; disease may be passed to child
Contraceptive use	Hormonal contraception may interrupt breastfeeding

for younger children in large families and may contribute to the economic well-being of the family, thus increasing both total family income and possibly per capita income.

Another hypothesis is that children who have a large number of siblings, regardless of their own birth order, are more likely to be in poor health. When there are a large number of children in a household with limited resources, there is increasing competition among children, so each child—not just children of higher birth order—may receive less time, attention, and care. Moreover, a child who has a larger number of siblings, especially if they live and sleep in crowded quarters, will be at increased risk of contracting infectious diseases.

Maternal Age

Children born to very young mothers and to older mothers may also be at higher risk of poor health and mortality. In the case of the children of very young mothers, as argued above, the reason may be that pregnancy is more stressful physiologically for adolescents because their reproductive systems are not yet fully mature, and they may not yet have completed their growth. As a consequence, adolescent girls may be less able to produce healthy babies and may experience more trauma during childbirth. A second possible reason that the children of very young mothers may be in poorer health is that these mothers may be less likely to seek and receive adequate prenatal care and may be less ready psychologically and materially to care for their children.

Children born to older mothers may also experience greater risks of mortality and morbidity. As argued above, women at the older end of the reproductive span may encounter more frequent problems during pregnancy and birth because the capability of their reproductive systems to cope with the burden of pregnancy has declined. Children born to older women may have poorer health at the time of birth because of the greater likelihood of birth trauma or genetic abnormalities.

Birth Spacing

Children born either after or before short interbirth intervals may also be at higher risk of morbidity and mortality, for several reasons. The first is related directly to the hypothesized effect of close pregnancy spacing on maternal health. For women living in poverty who are predisposed to malnutrition or poor health, a very short interval between one pregnancy and the next may not provide adequate time for rebuilding nutritional stores and for physiological recuperation. The consequences for children born after short interbirth intervals may be poorer intrauterine growth as well as a higher risk of preterm birth.

We noted above that competition among siblings in large families for scarce resources may mean that higher-order children, or possibly all children, may be at greater risk of poor health. Competition among children for family resources may be even more of a problem among children of similar ages, especially when they are young, because they have similar needs. When two births are spaced very closely, each child may not receive as much care and attention as he would if he did not have a sibling of roughly the same age. Close birth spacing can also create even more direct competition among siblings in the case of breastfeeding.

A mother who becomes pregnant soon after a child is born is likely to wean that child sooner than she would had she not become pregnant again. Since breastfeeding is an important determinant of child health in many societies, premature termination of breastfeeding often substantially increases a child's exposure to infection and increases the risk of malnutrition.

Close birth spacing may also increase children's exposure to infectious diseases by fostering transmission of infections among household members who are of similar ages. Many infectious childhood diseases affect a relatively narrow age range. If there is more than one child in the household in that age range, the chances of introducing the disease to the household and transmission of higher or repeated doses of the infectious organism may be dramatically increased, thus increasing the likelihood of multiple or more severe illnesses. This is especially a problem with diarrheal diseases, for which repeated incidence may result in malnutrition, and with measles, for which transmission in the household may be associated with more severe and fatal infection.

Unwanted Births

Finally, children who were unwanted at the time they were conceived may be at greater risk of poor health and mortality than other children. In households with limited resources, parents may, consciously or unconsciously, discriminate against unwanted children in the allocation of food, parental time and attention, or preventive and therapeutic health care. An alternative hypothesis is that children who are unwanted often are conceived when the family or the mother is under economic, social, or psychological stress, and the child is at greater risk simply by being born into a stressful situation.

Maternal Illness and Death and Effects on Child Health

Reproductive patterns may have another type of effect on the well-being of families and especially children, through their association with maternal morbidity and mortality. The death of a mother, whether due to reproductive or other causes, is likely to cause major disruption in the lives of her children, as well as a breakup of the household in which she and her children lived. In addition to the serious emotional consequences for children, the disruption following their mother's death may be extremely detrimental to their physical health, particularly if they are very young and breastfeeding has ended. Serious illness or reproductive injury may also prevent a woman from caring adequately for her children, with consequent negative effects on their health and survival chances. Maternal incapacity and death may be a growing burden on societies in which AIDS affects substantial numbers of women of reproductive age. Furthermore, it is possible that certain infectious diseases can be passed from mother to child.

INDIRECT EFFECTS OF REPRODUCTIVE PATTERNS ON HEALTH

Changes in reproductive patterns through control of fertility are also hypothesized to have important indirect effects on the health of women and children. Although some means of controlling fertility (including withdrawal and abstinence) are theoretically always available to couples, the availability of modern methods of contraception brings the process of fertility regulation more firmly into the control of couples and of women themselves. Successful intervention in what was formerly seen as a natural process may change couples' or families' attitudes about their ability to make changes in other traditional practices. These practices may include those related to child care, prenatal diet and care for women, and the use of modern health services. The ability to regulate fertility may also increase women's autonomy and give them greater authority to make decisions concerning their own health and the health of their children.

In some settings, increased control over fertility and the increased predictability of pregnancy timing that comes from contraceptive use may also make it easier for women to finish their education, to participate in the labor force, or to hold better-paying jobs. Higher educational attainment, work outside the home, or a better job are all likely to increase family income, which can then be spent on a more nutritious diet, better clothing and shelter, improvements in sanitation and water supply, and health services for all family members. In some societies, the fact that women make financial contributions to the household budget may also give them additional decision-making power in allocating household resources to themselves and their children, thus potentially improving their health.

Women who have fewer children or fewer young children to care for may be under substantially less physical and psychological stress than women with very large families, especially women in poor families, in which the resources to care for children are often scarce or inadequate. Furthermore, the ability to control fertility may also change a woman's outlook on life and may contribute to her psychological well-being (Dixon-Mueller, 1989).

In other settings, the ability to control fertility may create new tensions in the family, at least in the short run. The process of making explicit decisions about reproductive matters may lead to disagreement between spouses, conflicts between parents and their adult children about family size, and anxiety about violating traditional, often religious ideals surrounding sexual practices and childbearing.

Another hypothesized indirect effect of family planning on health relates to the use of health services. In countries where the program is strong and well-organized, family planning services may serve as an introduction for women to maternal and child health care services. Contact with family planning clinics may provide these women with information about how the health care system worked, referrals to other types of care, and often the confidence to deal with other types of health care workers. In other areas the opposite case may occur, with women being introduced to family planning through contact with the health care services.

OTHER POSSIBLE EXPLANATIONS

Reproductive patterns and women's and children's health may be associated with one another, without the former causing the latter, either directly or indirectly. A third factor may cause both. For example, a baby born after a pregnancy of short gestation is more likely to be in poor health and to be born within a short interval after the preceding birth. Although the short interval is not the cause of the child's poor health, both the short interval and the child's poorer health are due to the short gestation of the pregnancy. Or it is possible that the direction of causation runs from health to the reproductive pattern. For example, if a child dies shortly after birth, breastfeeding will be shorter than it otherwise would have been. As a consequence, postpartum amenorrhea (the infertile period following a birth, which is related to the duration and intensity of breastfeeding) will be shorter. Unless the couple compensates by practicing contraception longer than it would have had the child not died, the result will be a shorter birth interval. In this case, the birth interval is short because the child died.

All couples make implicit or explicit choices about whether or not to control their fertility, and, if they do decide to intervene, about how many children to have and when to have them. Decisions related to fertility control, family size, and birth spacing are unlikely to be entirely independent of women's and children's health or of other decisions people make which have consequences for their health. For example, a couple that experiences a child's death may choose to have another child to "replace" the one who died. Or when child mortality rates are high, couples may wish to "hedge" against the possibility of a child death by having additional births to increase the chances that a certain number of children will survive until maturity. Either of these mechanisms could result in a positive relationship between a large family and high child mortality, but, in these cases, fertility is high because mortality is high. A similar relationship could arise if some couples choose to have fewer children so that they can "invest" more in the health and education and material well-being of each child. In this case again, the relationship runs from (desired) health to fertility.

Another hypothesis about the observed association between fertility patterns and the health of women and children is that couples who use contraception to limit family size, space their children, and avoid unwanted pregnancies may simply be different from other couples in ways that affect both health and childbearing. An example of a couple's choices that affect both fertility and health involves the use of health services. As we noted above, in settings in which family planning programs are very strong, contact with family planning services may introduce families to other health services that they were previously unaware of. It is also possible that families who have previous experience with health services and are accustomed to using them are more likely to be aware of available family planning services and are also more likely to feel comfortable using them. Thus, it may be a familiarity with the health system that causes increased contraceptive use rather than vice versa.

Parents who take action to prevent illness and who seek medical care when illness occurs may also be more willing to attempt to control their fertility, to try using contraception, and to have the persistence to seek out contraceptive services when they are not readily available. Undertaking both health-related behavior and control of fertility may require a nonfatalistic view of life, in which it is possible and socially acceptable to try to intervene in natural processes such as illness and conception. For many couples in developing countries, obtaining effective health care and fertility control methods may require substantial persistence and knowledge of how to obtain information and deal with an ineffective delivery system. Adults who have these skills, abilities, and beliefs are likely to use health services, to carry out health-improving practices at home, and to use contraceptive services.

Finally, families with more financial resources and education are likely to be in better health—because they live in a better physical environment, because their diet is better, and because they receive better health care. These same families may also have fewer children because they prefer smaller families or because they have better access to contraceptive facilities.

In short, the observed association between reproductive patterns and women's and children's health may result from the fact that families who take measures to protect their members' health are also more likely to control their fertility, as well as from causal effects of reproductive patterns on health. This possibility is important to consider if we want to determine the likely effects of changes in reproductive patterns on health, and we return to it in subsequent chapters.

AVAILABLE EVIDENCE

Probably the most direct and convincing way to distinguish among the hypotheses discussed above would be to conduct controlled randomized double-blind experiments. For example, some women would be randomly assigned to have their first child at age 16 and others would wait till age 20. Or two otherwise identical sets of communities could be chosen for study and contraception would be provided in one group and not the other. Such experiments, however, are difficult to perform, and they would raise ethical problems even if they were feasible. Consequently, it is not surprising that the extant evidence is based not on experimental studies, but rather on observational data collected through surveys or longitudinal data from nonexperimental settings.

For policy purposes, we would like to be able to distinguish among the alternative hypotheses discussed above. To illustrate, take the example of the relationship between young maternal age and child health. If the reason that the children of teenagers are less healthy than the children of older women is that teenagers are less likely to seek prenatal care, further research could seek to understand the reasons and to try to remedy the situation. If the relationship between young maternal age and child health is physiological, due to incomplete maternal growth, a policy that helps women postpone childbearing until later ages should result in improved child health. If, alternatively, teenage mothers have poorer child health outcomes because girls who become pregnant as teenagers are poorer mothers regardless of the ages at which they bear their children, then postponing childbearing for these women will not necessarily have beneficial effects for the children's health. A key question is whether teenagers outgrow— physiologically, psychologically, or economically—whatever causes their children to have poorer health outcomes, or whether it is a persistent characteristic of the types of women who become pregnant as teenagers.

The evidence regarding the hypothesized effect of maternal age on children's health typically comes from analyses of data on maternal ages at children's births and the children's health (typically survival measures) that show health outcomes to be poorer for children born to young mothers under age 20 than to older mothers ages 20-29. Earlier studies tended to consider the simple correlation between maternal age and child health. Such a correlation, however, says nothing about which among the possible mechanisms discussed in this chapter might account for this association. For example, births to teenage mothers are more likely than births to older mothers to be first-order births, which have a greater risk of low birthweight and other problems, as discussed above. Hence, to assess the effect of being born to a teenage mother, it is important to hold constant the effect of parity and, in essence, consider age differentials within parity categories. As another example, teenage mothers may have less education or lower incomes than older mothers. In such a case, it is desirable to control for education and income, so as not to attribute to age what is really a result of low education or income. More recent studies have used multivariate statistical methods in an attempt to deal with these issues.

The remaining possibilities are more difficult to distinguish, especially in large-scale population surveys, which have provided much of the evidence on the relationships between reproductive patterns and child health. To assess the possibility of a physiological mechanism, one would ideally like to consider gynecological age (years since menarche) and assess its relation to pelvic size and the women's nutritional status, and how these, in turn, affect her baby's health. Psychological maturity is even more difficult to assess; for example, teenagers tend to be more egocentric than older women and less likely to respond to the needs of others. One could look at the health-related behaviors that psychological development could be expected to affect, to see, for example, if pregnant teenagers are less likely to use prenatal care (appropriately). However, assessing the effects of health care on health outcomes is complicated by the fact that unobserved factors that affect decisions to seek health care may also affect health outcomes. For example, as noted above, women with a greater concern about health may be both more likely to seek health care and more likely to engage in other behaviors that promote good health. In such a case, a simple correlation between health care and health would overstate the direct effect of the former on the latter. In other cases, women in poor health may be more likely to seek health care because of specific needs.

The last example illustrates a problem generic to all research that uses nonexperimental observational data: no matter how many known correlates and potential confounding variables are controlled (e.g., parity, education, and income in assessing the effect of young maternal age on child health), it is always possible that there may be unobserved factors that may be correlated with both the reproductive patterns of interest and the health outcome being considered that contribute to their relationship; hence, even when other observed factors are controlled, it is possible that the estimated relationship is not entirely causal. Some analysts have used structural models to deal with these issues, but to date such methods have been used infrequently to study the effects of reproductive patterns on women's and children's health, particularly in developing countries.

An example of using structural models is the simultaneous equation framework as commonly used in economics, for example, when fertility is modified in response to the expectation and occurrence of child mortality, while child mortality may be affected by reproductive patterns. To disentangle the two effects, which operate in opposite directions, and to statistically distinguish only the latter effect, which is one focus of this report, the scientist requires information on an independent variable that directly affects fertility and does not directly affect child mortality. This variable could provide the information needed to identify statistically and thus estimate the one-way effect of independent changes in reproductive patterns on child (or maternal) mortality. The problem is to find such an identifying variable that can be plausibly excluded from entering the mortality determining process. This is difficult when studying complex, jointly determined household demographic processes such as fertility and child mortality, especially when the assumptions made in choosing identifying variables are often unverifiable.

The evidence reviewed in this report comes from many different sources: large-scale population-based surveys that ask women about their pregnancies and children's mortality, smaller-scale longitudinal studies and hospital or clinic samples that often include physiological information, and data on births and deaths in historical populations. The characteristics and advantages and disadvantages of these various types of studies are reviewed in the chapters ahead. However, it is important to note that none of the studies to date has simultaneously addressed all the different types of issues just discussed.

This report focuses principally on the evidence from previous research concerning the hypotheses about the direct effects of family planning or reproductive control on the health of women and children. Although it is possible that indirect effects may be equally or more important than the direct effects under consideration, investigation of these hypotheses is outside the scope of this report. We return to the subject of the indirect effects in Chapter 7.

3

Reproductive Patterns and Women's Health

In comparison with the levels in industrialized countries, reproductive mortality remains high in most developing countries, particularly in rural areas. In developing countries, maternal mortality is estimated to range from approximately 100 to 700 or more maternal deaths per 100,000 live births, with the highest levels in rural areas of sub-Saharan Africa and South Asia. These rates imply an estimated 500,000 maternal deaths annually, with over 98 percent occurring in developing countries (World Health Organization, 1985b). In industrialized countries, maternal mortality was at about that same level at the turn of the century but has declined to a current level of less than 10 maternal deaths per 100,000 live births, with under 10,000 deaths per year. Thus, although a majority of pregnancies proceed normally and are not associated with significant health problems, there remains considerable potential for reducing the risks associated with pregnancy and childbearing.

The most important causes of reproductive injury, morbidity, and mortality in developing countries are obstructed labor (and ruptured uterus), postpartum hemorrhage, pregnancy-induced hypertension, postpartum infection, and the complications of unsafe abortion. The relative importance of each of these causes varies among populations and within the same country, depending on living conditions and the availability of medical care.

In this chapter, we summarize the evidence concerning the relation between reproductive patterns and women's health. As described in Chapter 2, there are at least two ways in which changes in reproductive patterns may improve women's health. First, each time a woman becomes pregnant or gives birth, she is susceptible to an increased risk of illness, injury, or mortality that she does not face when she is not pregnant. Women who have more pregnancies or give birth to more children encounter this basic risk more frequently than women with lower fertility. Thus, a reduction in the number of pregnancies or births that women have will improve their reproductive health simply by reducing the frequency of exposure to the basic risk of illness, injury, and mortality associated with pregnancy and childbirth.

Second, women experiencing certain types of pregnancies undergo an additional risk. As described in Chapter 2, it has been hypothesized that higher-risk pregnancies include:

- first pregnancies or births, pregnancies of young women, or the combination;
- pregnancies in women at high parity, pregnancies of older women, or the combination;
- pregnancies following soon after previous pregnancies; and
- pregnancies that are terminated by unsafe induced abortion.

The effects of these higher-risk pregnancies are the focus of much of this chapter. However, before reviewing this research, we discuss the types of evidence on which our conclusions about the associations between women's health and reproductive patterns are based.

SOURCES OF EVIDENCE

Measurement and Data

There are two standard measures of the frequency of maternal death in a population. The first is the *maternal mortality ratio*, which is the ratio of the number of deaths due to pregnancy or childbirth to the number of pregnancies. However, in practice, even in an industrialized country, it is impossible to count the total number of pregnancies. Thus, by convention, the number of live births is used as the denominator.

The second measure is the *maternal mortality rate* or the maternal cause-specific mortality rate, which is calculated by dividing the number of deaths due to pregnancy and childbirth by the number of women of reproductive ages. Unfortunately, these two measures are often used interchangeably in the public health literature, and reports of rates often are actually referring to ratios. For clarity, in this report the denominator (either women or live births) is always stated explicitly.

Information on levels of maternal mortality and other indices of reproductive health is difficult to obtain, especially in developing countries. It is even more difficult to obtain data adequate to investigate the possible associations between reproductive patterns and maternal health. There are several reasons for the paucity of data on levels and trends in maternal mortality. First, vital registration in most developing countries is seriously incomplete: relatively few deaths, especially in rural areas, are registered. In addition, deaths occurring very early in pregnancy (such as those caused by ectopic pregnancies), those caused by complications of induced abortion, and those attributed to other causes (such as malaria and hepatitis) are often not classified as due to reproductive causes. Even in industrialized countries where the numbers of births and deaths are known, causes of maternal death are not well reported. The majority of studies discussed in this chapter define maternal mortality as a pregnancy-related death, due to either direct causes (pregnancy complications) or indirect causes (other diseases such as heart disease exacerbated by pregnancy).

Poor vital registration is a problem that affects the availability of data on infant and child mortality as well as maternal mortality. However, in the case of infant and child mortality, vital registration data can be supplemented by levels and associated risk factors from national or local fertility surveys or from field studies in small areas in which data are collected over time. Data on maternal mortality, by contrast, are considerably more difficult to obtain from these two sources (Zimicki, 1989). Reproductive histories and histories of child death are usually collected from women, but maternal mortality data are difficult to collect in this way, since women who died cannot be interviewed, and collecting data on the reproductive histories of decedents from other sources is difficult. The Demographic and Health Survey Project plans to test an indirect method of obtaining maternal mortality estimates asking adults in households if they had a sister who died shortly before or after childbirth.

Measuring maternal mortality of entire populations in developing countries is also difficult because death from reproductive causes remains a relatively rare event. For example, maternal mortality ratios of 700 deaths per 100,000 live births have been reported in some parts of Africa. But even with these high levels of death, a sample of 100,000 women would be necessary to yield 700 maternal deaths. By contrast, in these same populations, current levels of infant mortality rates imply that there will be between 10,000 and 20,000 infant deaths per 100,000 live births. Since maternal death is a relatively rare event, accurate measurement of maternal mortality rates requires collecting data from a much larger population than would be required for accurate measurement of infant and child mortality. The problem of sample size is somewhat smaller in the case of illnesses associated with pregnancy, since maternal morbidity is more common than mortality. However, since morbidity is a less well-defined event than mortality, it tends to be even more poorly reported. Thus, information with which to evaluate the association between reproduction patterns and maternal illness or mortality generally is not available, because data on both maternal illness or mortality and on reproductive history are required for a very large population.

This report draws on studies of the association between maternal health and reproductive patterns that are based on three sources of data: general population-based studies, hospital-population studies, and hospital case series.

Population-based studies allow nearly complete counts of live births and maternal deaths, although they suffer from the same types of underestimation as vital registration systems. Very few population-based studies concerning maternal mortality in developing countries have been published: four from Bangladesh (Chen et al., 1975; Khan et al., 1986; Alauddin, 1987; Koenig et al., 1988a), one from Ethiopia (Kwast et al., 1986), one from Egypt (Fortney et al., 1985), one from Gambia (Greenwood et al., 1987), and one from Jamaica (Walker et al., 1985). Preliminary results from population-based studies in India (Bhatia, 1985) and Bangladesh (Lindpaintner et al., 1982) are available. In addition, one hospital-based study from Lusaka, Zambia (Mhango et al., 1986), arguably covers a sufficient proportion of the population (85 percent of births, 90 percent of deaths) to be considered a population-based study. However, the number of deaths in each study is relatively small, so estimates for subgroups of women with particular characteristics are unstable. Characteristics of the data and types of analysis used in these and the studies cited are presented at the end of this chapter in Appendix Table 3.A.

Studies of hospital patients, particularly those carried out in referral hospitals, provide less accurate estimates of the incidence of maternal mortality or morbidity than population-based studies. There are several reasons to expect that maternal mortality ratios from hospital studies are unrepresentative. First, hospital patient studies reflect the experience of only a proportion of the population during only part of the risk period—usually at the time of or immediately after the pregnancy outcome. Thus, deaths occurring outside the hospital and those occurring some time before and after delivery and discharge are usually missed. Second, rural women are likely to be underrepresented in such studies. For example, a woman living in a rural area with an ectopic pregnancy or one who has postpartum hemorrhage is likely to die before she can reach a hospital. In addition, cause-specific mortality measures may be affected by the types of complications that allow time for a woman to be moved to a hospital. Third, the population delivering in hospitals on a nonemergency basis represents a more socioeconomically advantaged portion of the population and is likely to have had greater-than-average exposure to prenatal care. Finally, since most women in developing countries do not deliver in hospitals but may be brought there on an emergency basis if the delivery is complicated, hospital populations tend to have more abnormal or complicated cases. Thus, hospital data are likely to overestimate maternal mortality ratios and provide a misleading picture of maternal morbidity.

Even if national maternal mortality ratios cannot be accurately estimated with hospital data, if the assumption can be made that deaths in hospitals are representative of all maternal deaths, or if the way in which they are unrepresentative can be identified, then cause-specific mortality rates from these sources may be useful. Because of the very small numbers of deaths identified in population-based studies, hospital-based studies provide valuable sources of data for examining the causes of high maternal mortality.

Case series studies are based on reports about a series of deaths, which could be deaths from all maternal causes or from a specific cause, such as ruptured uterus. These series can provide information about case-fatality rates. Unfortunately, most case studies contain no description of the population from which the cases are drawn. Thus, they do not provide evidence on the level of maternal mortality or the influence of reproductive patterns on women's health.

Methodological Issues

Aside from problems associated with the available data, studies of the association between reproductive patterns and maternal health are more limited than those available on child health for two methodological reasons. First, few of the available studies use multivariate statistical techniques to control for potentially confounding variables (see Appendix Table 3.A), as do most of the studies of child health on which we draw. Thus, it is more difficult to conclude that specific high-risk characteristics are causally related to maternal mortality. For example, poor women both may have more births (and thus achieve higher parity) and may be less likely to obtain adequate interpartum care. This could result in an upward bias in the estimated effect of high parity on maternal morbidity and mortality.

Second, many studies of maternal health fail to hold constant the effects of other reproductive variables. For example, the association of poor pregnancy outcome and births to teenagers may be partly due to the fact that many of these births are first births.

EFFECTS OF YOUNG MATERNAL AGE AND PRIMIPARITY

Most studies of pregnancy complications or maternal mortality have investigated their association with either young maternal age or first parity, but not with both. Because age and parity are strongly associated, it is often unclear whether the age-specific and parity-specific patterns reflect the same basic risks based on parity, whether they have independent effects, or whether they act in combination. An answer to this question would require more studies of maternal mortality that control for age and parity simultaneously, but few such studies are available (see Koenig et al., 1988a; Walker et al., 1985).

Both population-based and hospital studies indicate that the first pregnancy is strongly associated with a higher risk of maternal mortality. For example, population-based studies from Bangladesh, Ethiopia, and Gambia indicate that the risk of maternal mortality is up to three times higher for the first birth than for subsequent births. Also, in developed countries and in some developing countries, such as Jamaica, where the possibility of death associated with any birth is much lower than in Africa or South Asia, there is also a higher risk associated with the first birth.

There is conflicting evidence about whether pregnancies at maternal ages below 20 are inherently riskier than pregnancies at ages 20 through 24. The largest population-based study, with 14,631 first births (Koenig et al., 1988a), shows no increased risk, though smaller studies from the same area (Chen etØal., 1975) and from Indonesia (Chi et al., 1981) and Jamaica (Walker et al., 1985) indicate a slightly elevated risk of death. A significant problem with these studies, however, is that all births to women under 20 are combined in recent studies. There is evidence that the increase in risks is most important for young women under age 17, particularly those under 15. For example, a hospital study in Nigeria showed that the risk of mortality varied inversely with age, with women 15 or younger having 10 times, 16-year-olds 4 times, and 17-19-year-olds twice the risk of those ages 20-24 (Harrison and Rossiter, 1985). In Tanzania there were 2-3 times more deaths during their first pregnancy or birth among the younger women (Arkutu, 1978). The possibility that this pattern is influenced by selection bias cannot be ruled out, however, since younger women may be less likely to be brought to hospitals unless they have serious complications (Harrison and Rossiter, 1985).

Studies in both developed and developing countries that have considered causes of morbidity or mortality in younger and primigravid women indicate that pregnancy-induced hypertension is most common among women during their first pregnancies and more common among younger women (Arkutu, 1978; Efiong and Banjoko, 1975; Faundes et al., 1974; World Health Organization, 1988). Obstructed labor because of the pelvis's being too small to allow the child's head to pass is most common in young primigravid women (Aitken and Walls, 1986). Malaria is more frequent and the infection appears to be heavier during first, and to a certain extent, second pregnancies, than during later pregnancies (McGregor et al., 1983).

The increased risk for younger primigravidas may reflect not so much increased physiological risk as socioeconomic differences between the younger mothers and women who have their first child at ages 20-24. For example, women who have their first child earlier may be from poorer families (Efiong and Banjoko, 1975) and have less access to or make less use of prenatal care than those who have their first child after age 20 (Jelley and Madeley, 1983).

EFFECTS OF OLDER MATERNAL AGE, HIGH PARITY, OR BOTH

The problem of confounding between age and parity exists as well for births to older women, which are in most cases also high-order births. A pattern of generally increasing risk of maternal death with each successive birth after the second or third birth is evident in the information from three population studies. Women of parity 5 or more have about 1.5 to 3 times the risk of maternal death than women at the lowest-risk parities (2 and 3). In general, within any parity, older women, particularly those over age 35, tend to be at higher risk of death (Koenig et al., 1988a; Chi et al., 1981; Walker et al., 1985).

Older, multiparous women are more likely to have problems with malpresentation, in which the fetus lies in a position other than in the usual head first position (a breech or transverse lie, for example). Malpresentation may occur because the muscles of the uterine wall become flaccid with repeated stretching of successive pregnancies. The condition can result in uterine rupture, hemorrhage associated with rupture, or with unsuccessful attempts to remedy the situation (such as the excessive use of oxytocin-containing medicine, abdominal pressure on the uterus, or manipulation of the fetus) and infection.

Another cause of hemorrhage is placental abnormality. Faundes et al. (1974) found an abnormal placenta to be more common in women above age 35 and in women who had had 5 or more previous births. Antepartum hemorrhage can arise from several causes, the most important being placenta previa (a condition occurring when the placenta overlies the cervical opening of the uterus, resulting in massive, fatal hemorrhage at the time of attempted delivery unless a cesarian section is performed) and abruptia placenta (a condition occurring when the placenta separates prematurely from the uterus prior to delivery of the baby), which if untreated leads to fetal death, hemorrhage, and blood clotting. Postpartum hemorrhage, which is the most common complication among high-parity women, arises primarily from uterine atony (or lack of contraction of uterine muscles), sometimes secondary to a retained placenta (a condition in which the placenta is not expelled after delivery of the baby).

EFFECTS OF SHORT INTERVALS BETWEEN BIRTHS

Although a number of researchers have hypothesized what is called a maternal depletion effect of short interbirth intervals that would increase the risk of maternal mortality (Jelliffe, 1976; Omran and Standley, 1981; Rinehart and Kols, 1984; Winikoff, 1983), no study yet identified has specifically addressed the issue of the relationship between birth interval length and maternal mortality in developing countries.

There is indirect evidence from Matlab, Bangladesh, suggesting that short intervals are not associated with a higher risk of maternal mortality: for each 5-year age group of women, the risk of mortality decreased with increasing parity, at least through parity 6 (Koenig et al., 1988a). Among women of the same age, those of higher parity will, on average, have had shorter birth intervals. Thus, this study seems to suggest that women with the shortest birth intervals are least likely to die. The reason, however, could be due to selection: the healthiest women may become pregnant more quickly and therefore achieve higher parities.

EFFECTS OF PREGNANCY IN INCREASING MORTALITY FROM OTHER CONDITIONS

Pregnancy increases the likelihood that a woman will die of certain conditions (i.e., case-fatality rates are increased). These conditions include chronic illnesses that antedate the pregnancy, such as rheumatic heart disease, diabetes, sickle-cell disease and AIDS, as well as acute infectious diseases that the woman contracts while pregnant. Examples of these acutely infectious diseases are hepatitis and epidemic malaria, for which case-fatality rates are higher for pregnant than for nonpregnant women (Morrow et al., 1968). More generally, women who are malnourished or in poor health may be more likely to experience problems during a pregnancy. This is particularly true for women who are severely anemic.

EFFECTS OF UNSAFE INDUCED ABORTION

In countries where safe abortion is not available, many women suffer serious complications and often death as a consequence of unsafe abortion procedures. Unsafe abortion can cause uterine perforation, hemorrhage, uterine and generalized infection, acute bleeding disorders, and embolism to the lung and brain.

Kwast et al. (1986) report that postabortion complications are the most common cause of maternal mortality in Addis Ababa, Ethiopia, especially among primigravid, unmarried women employed as domestics and students. Koenig et al. (1988a) attribute 18 percent of maternal mortality in Matlab Thana, Bangladesh, to postabortion complications.

Additional insights into the health consequences of unsafe abortion can be derived from the experience in Romania, where restrictive abortion laws were enacted after a history of relatively liberal laws, resulting in a sevenfold increase in maternal mortality due to abortion (Tietze, 1983). At the same time, data from the United States demonstrates the extremely low risk of safe, first-trimester abortion procedures, making them one of the safest surgical procedures performed.

CONCLUSION

A reduction in the number of pregnancies and births that a woman experiences enables her to unambiguously reduce her risk of reproductive complications and maternal mortality merely by reducing the number of times she is exposed to that risk. While there are potential risks to using contraception, the research reviewed in the next chapter demonstrates that the risks a woman assumes in using contraception are very small compared with the health benefits of reducing exposure to pregnancy and birth-related health problems. Moreover, some contraceptives have noncontraceptive health benefits (see Chapter 4).

Data from Bangladesh show declines in the maternal mortality rate (per 100,000 women) associated with reduction in fertility (Koenig et al., 1988a). Other evidence presented in this chapter indicates that certain changes in reproductive patterns may also be beneficial to women's health, over and above the effect of reducing the absolute number of births women have. The basic pattern observed for the relationship between fertility and maternal mortality is that risk of mortality is highest for first pregnancies and for fifth and subsequent pregnancies. This pattern exists whatever the overall level of maternal mortality, but, as conditions improve, the U-shaped curve of risk with parity is not only lower, but also flatter. Extremes of age, lack of medical care, poverty, and some infectious diseases also increase the risk. However, no studies have shown a reduction in the maternal mortality ratio (per 100,000 live births) as a result of changes in age or parity distributions of births.

For first births, particularly among young women, use of contraception can reduce maternal mortality by delaying first births until after age 20 or by reducing the number of unwanted pregnancies that might otherwise result in abortion. However, teenagers may not use contraception effectively, resulting in excessive use of abortion as a means of preventing unwanted births. This is not inevitable, however, as shown by the experience in Canada and Scandinavian countries, where more effective sex education efforts and easier access to contraception resulted in declines of both pregnancies and abortions among young women (Tietze, 1983; Henshaw, 1986). Clearly, where safe abortions are not available, effective family planning use by teenagers is even more important as a means of reducing mortality associated with unwanted first births.

Evidence presented in this chapter suggests that changing reproductive patterns can reduce the maternal mortality rate (per 100,000 women) by:

- reducing the total number of pregnancies each woman has in lifetime;
- reducing the incidence of high-risk pregnancies (high parity, very young maternal age and older maternal age, pregnancy among women with major health problems (e.g., hypertension, diabetes, heart disease, and malaria); and
- reducing the demand for abortion to terminate unwanted pregnancies in countries where safe abortion is unavailable.

APPENDIX TABLE 3.A Summary of Studies of Maternal Health

Study	Location	Measures of Maternal Condition	Tabulation Variables
POPULATION-BASED STUDIES			
Alauddin, 1987	Bangladesh	Maternal mortality ratio[1]	Age, parity, landholding, economic status, education, gravidity
Bhatia, 1985	India	Maternal deaths	Age, rural/urban, parity
Chen, Gesche, Ahmed, Chowdhury and Moseley, 1975	Bangladesh	Maternal mortality ratio[1]	Age, parity, living children, gravidity

34   *CONTRACEPTION AND REPRODUCTION*

APPENDIX TABLE 3.A Continued

Study	Location	Measures of Maternal Condition	Tabulation Variables
Fortney, Susanti, Gadalla, Saleh, Feldblum, and Potts, 1985	Egypt, Indonesia	Total deaths, maternal deaths, maternal mortality, rate[2] and ratio[1]	Cause of death, age
Greenwood, Greenwood, Bradley, Williams, Shenton, Tulloch, Byass and Oldfield, 1987	Rural Gambia	Maternal mortality ratio[1]	Age, parity, prenatal visits, attendant, cause of death, place of delivery, place of death, time of death relative to delivery, pregnancy outcome
Khan, Jahan and Begum, 1986	Bangladesh	Maternal mortality ratio[1]	Age, parity, place, cause of death, attendant
Koenig, Fauveau, Chowdhury, Chakraborty, and Khan, 1988	Bangladesh	Maternal mortality rate[2] and ratio, maternal deaths, total deaths	Age, parity, gravidity, year
Kwast, Rochat, Kidane-Mariam, 1986	Ethiopia	Maternal deaths, maternal mortality ratio[1]	Age, parity, education, marital status, income, prenatal care, occupation, wantedness of pregnancy
Lindpainter, Jahan, Satterthwaite, and Zimicki, 1982	Bangladesh	Maternal deaths, maternal mortality ratio[1]	Age, gravidity, cause of death, area
Walker, Ashley, McCaw and Bernard, 1985	Jamaica	Maternal deaths, maternal mortality ratio[1]	Cause of death, time relative to delivery, age, parity

- -

HOSPITAL AND CLINIC-BASED STUDIES

Aitken and Walls, 1986	Sierra Leone	Cephalopelvic dispositions and primigravidas (size of the fetal head in relation to the maternal pelvis of women pregnant for the first time)	Maternal height

APPENDIX TABLE 3.A Continued

Study	Location	Measures of Maternal Condition	Tabulation Variables
Arkutu, 1978	Tanzania	Primigravidas (women pregnant for the first time)	Complications, mode of delivery, duration of labor, age, birthwight
Chi, Agoestina, and Harbin, 1981	Indonesia	Maternal deaths maternal mortality ratio[1]	Cause of death, underlying condition, age, parity, urban/rural admission, anemic/not, hospital
Efiong and Banjoko, 1975	Nigeria	Comparison of very young and old primigravid women	Income class, height, prenatal complication, duration of labor, mode of delivery, blood loss, birthweight
Faundes, Fanjul, Henriquez, Mora, and Tognola, 1974	Chile	Deliveries, neonatal mortality	Hypertension, ampresentation, placental hemorrhage, congenital malformation parity, postpartum hemorrhage
Harrison and Rossiter, 1985	Nigeria	Maternal deaths, pregnancies, maternal mortality ratio[1]	duration in hospital, ethnicity, residence, religion, education, parity, age
Jelley and Madely, 1983	Mozambigue	Information from prenatal clinic forms	Age, health center, category, attendants
McGregor, Wilson, and Billewicz, 1983	Gambia	Deliveries	Placental parasitemia, area, urban/rural, parity, sex,
Mhango, Rochat, and Arkutu, 1986	Zambia	Births, maternal deaths, maternal mortality	Age, parity, cause-specific, type of prenatal care; Case reports: cause of death, parity, marital status, socioeconomic status, time relative to delivery
Morrow, Smetana, Sai and Edscomb, 1968	Ghana	Hepatitis patients, including pregnant and postpartum females	Coma status, pregnancy status, sex, age

[1] Deaths due to pregnancy or childbirth per 100,000 live births.

[2] Deaths due to pregnancy or childbirth per 100,000 women of reproductive ages.

4

Contraceptive Benefits and Risks

Pregnancy and childbirth carry risks of morbidity and mortality. Although the contraceptives that couples use to avoid pregnancy have their own health risks, they also have substantial noncontraceptive health benefits. Information about these risks and benefits is necessary for informed decision making. Oral contraceptives, for example, not only prevent pregnancy, but they also reduce the risk of endometrial and ovarian cancer and protect against acute pelvic inflammatory disease and ectopic pregnancies. However, oral contraceptives increase the risk of cardiovascular disease. IUDs provide effective contraception but increase the potential for infection in certain high-risk groups. Barrier methods of contraception provide less effective contraception, but they protect against sexually transmitted infections including human immunodeficiency virus (HIV). The importance of the noncontraceptive benefits and risks of contraceptives varies among societies because of variations in the prevalence of the diseases involved.

This chapter reviews evidence on the effectiveness and health consequences of specific contraceptive methods. Our attention is limited to the biological consequences of a method's use, even though each method may have psychological risks and benefits. Our purpose is to provide an account of the direct health consequences of contraceptive use, independent of the effects that fertility control has on health by allowing women to control their fertility. This analysis is particularly important because, in some countries, health officials downplay the health benefits of lower fertility because they fear the adverse health effects of widespread use of modern contraceptives, especially in circumstances in which medical supervision of contraceptive practice is limited.

36

Our consideration of the effectiveness of contraceptives is based on a recent critical review of the literature by Trussell and Kost (1987). The studies they examined and most of the epidemiologic and clinical studies of the health effects of contraceptives have been carried out in developed countries. We recognize the difficulty of generalizing these results to the special health and cultural situations in the developing world. Furthermore, there are few studies of the effects of various contraceptive methods on the risk of diseases that are generally limited to developing countries. In many cases, the available data pertain to contraceptives that were commonly used in the 1960s and early 1970s and focus on the user population at that time. The research design, the quality of the data, the size of the sample, and the analysis have often been insufficient to allow definitive conclusions. Clearly, more studies conducted in developing countries are needed, and in fact studies sponsored by the World Health Organization are under way. Nevertheless, we regard the available information as a reasonable guide for estimating the risk of pregnancy versus the risks and benefits of contraceptive use in the developing world.

ORAL CONTRACEPTIVES

According to United Nations estimates, oral contraceptives are currently used by nearly 62 million women (United Nations, 1989). Two types of oral contraceptives (OCs) are available: combination OCs, consisting of the hormones estrogen and progestin, and the progestin-only pill (often called the minipill). Combination OCs are used by far more women, and as a result, most epidemiologic studies consider this type, particularly the formulations popular during the 1960s to mid-1970s. OCs prevent pregnancy primarily by inhibiting ovulation, although changes in the cervical mucous and endometrium may also have contraceptive effects. Failure rates associated with OC use are low—roughly 3 percent of women using OCs became pregnant in the first year of use, mainly because of improper or incomplete use (Trussell and Kost, 1987).

Health Benefits

A large cohort study in the United Kingdom has provided clear evidence that OC use decreases the risk of iron deficiency anemia in both current and past users (Royal College of General Practitioners, 1970). The effect is probably caused by the decrease in menstrual flow and consequent increase in iron reserves. This benefit may be especially important in developing countries in which iron deficiency is a problem (Stadel, 1986).

Case-control and cohort studies have found a decreased risk of benign breast disease associated with OC use (Stadel, 1986). The relative risk in women who have used OCs for more than two years compared with nonusers is about 0.6 for fibrocystic disease, 0.3 for fibroadenoma, and about 0.5 for unbiopsied breast lumps. This decreased risk does not persist in former users who have not used OCs for more than one year (Brinton et al., 1981). Since this effect is most likely to be related to the high progestin content of early formulations of the pill, current OC formulations may not decrease the risk of benign breast disease.

Several studies have found that OC use decreases the risk of functional ovarian cysts. This effect is probably due to the suppression of ovulation (Stadel, 1986). Evidence also suggests that OCs protect against uterine fibroids, the protection increasing with the duration of OC use (Ross et al., 1986). While there is still speculation about the mechanism, the protective effect against fibroids may be related to how the effect of circulating estrogens, which may promote the formation of fibroids, is modified by the progestins in OCs.

Several studies in developed and developing countries have found that current or recent OC use reduces the risk of pelvic inflammatory disease (PID), a major cause of female infertility (Stadel, 1986; Gray and Campbell, 1985). These studies have found that OC use lowers the risk by, on average, about 40 percent. Two mechanisms may be operative: OCs may change the cervical mucous such that it prevents pathogenic organisms from ascending into the upper genital tract; or OCs reduce menstrual blood flow, thus decreasing the amount of medium available for bacterial growth (Rubin et al., 1982). Unfortunately, most of the studies of oral contraceptives and PID have been hospital-based, so the results may not apply to women who are asymptomatic or who have PID not requiring hospitalization (Washington et al., 1985). For example, OCs may protect against gonorrhea, an important cause of acute PID that would require hospitalization, whereas other bacterial etiologies that cause less severe PID, such as chlamydia, may receive little or no protection from OC use.

Because they are highly effective at inhibiting ovulation, OCs greatly decrease the risk of ectopic pregnancy. Results from large case-control studies conducted in the United States and developing countries found that current OC users were 10 times less likely to have an ectopic pregnancy than women using no method (Ory and the Women's Health Study, 1981; Gray, 1984). Because the risk of death from ectopic pregnancy is high for women living in rural areas in the developing world, this effect is particularly noteworthy.

Another important benefit from OC use is a reduction in the risk of endometrial and ovarian cancer. Several epidemiologic studies have confirmed reduction of endometrial cancer among users. The Cancer and Steroid Hormone (CASH) study conducted in the United States found a 40 percent reduction in the risk of endometrial cancer, even long after OC use had been discontinued, and the benefit increased with the cumulative duration of pill use (Centers for Disease Control and the National Institute of Child Health and Human Development, 1987a, 1987b). The continued protection the pill provides to former users is not clearly understood, but apparently the carcinogenic effect of estrogen on the endometrium is obviated by the progestin in the pill.

The CASH study also found a 40 percent reduction in the risk of ovarian cancer (Centers for Disease Control and National Institute of Child Health and Human Development, 1987a, 1987b). Other epidemiologic studies have supported these findings. Suppression of ovulation and suppression of secretion of the hormone gonadotropin have both been postulated as mechanisms of this protection. It is noteworthy that there is consistent evidence from independent epidemiologic studies that the pill protects women from endometrial and ovarian cancer. Such consistency suggests true biological effect.

Adverse Health Effects: Cardiovascular Diseases

Cardiovascular diseases are a major cause of death in developed countries, where most research on the association between OC use and cardiovascular diseases has been conducted. These diseases are less common in developing countries, so alteration in their occurrence by OC use may not be as substantial as in industrialized countries.

OC use increases the risk of cardiovascular disease, in particular the risk of venous thromboembolism, myocardial infarction, and stroke (Stadel, 1986; Prentice and Thomas, 1987; Vessey, 1980). The risk of serious illness or death attributable to OC use from adverse cardiovascular effects is concentrated primarily among older women over age 30 and women who smoke cigarettes or have other cardiovascular risk factors. The excess risk of cardiovascular diseases seems to be directly related to both the estrogen and progestin content of the pill. And the risks may be substantially lower with newer low-dose preparations.

Venous thrombosis is the blockage of a vein by a blood clot particle. Thromboembolism occurs when the blood clot moves from a primary site to another, such as to the lungs or the brain. It is a major source of illness that may lead to death. Although the risk of venous thromboembolism is increased for current OC users, the increased risk does not persist among former users and is not related to duration of use (Vessey, 1980). The higher the estrogen content of the OC, the greater is the risk of venous thromboembolism, both for superficial and deep vein thrombosis (Stadel, 1986). The risk of venous thromboembolism among pill users appears to be unrelated to cigarette smoking. Mechanisms underlying increases in venous thromboembolism involve effects of estrogen or blood clotting factors that increase the coagulability of blood.

Myocardial infarction and stroke are much more important causes of mortality attributable to OCs. The risk is strongly influenced by age and by the presence of other cardiovascular risk factors, including cigarette smoking, hypertension, and diabetes. The annual risk of myocardial infarction attributable to current OC use rises from about 4 cases per 100,000 among nonsmoking OC users ages 30 to 39 to 185 cases per 100,000 among heavy-smoking OC users ages 40 to 44 (Stadel, 1986). Current OC use has been found to slightly elevate blood pressure in most women, possibly a contributing factor to the pathogenesis of myocardial infarction and stroke among current OC users. OC use leads to a three- to sixfold increase in the risk of overt hypertension, increasing with a woman's age and duration of OC use. It must be remembered that these risks pertain to use of the relatively high-dose pills of the 1960s and 1970s and their patterns of use in relation to such factors as age and smoking.

Other Possible Health Effects

Metabolic Effects

Metabolic changes may underlie the effects of OCs on myocardial infarction. Estrogens have the apparently desirable effect of increasing HDL-cholesterol (high density lipoprotein) concentration. Depending on type, progestins may either increase, decrease, or have no effect on HDL-cholesterol (for a complete discussion of changes in HDL-cholesterol, see Vessey, 1980). The net effect of different OC formulations on HDL-cholesterol is a function of both the dose of estrogen and the dose and type of progestin (Stadel, 1986).

Current OC use has been found to decrease glucose tolerance in most women, although this decrease appears to be small and unrelated to duration of use. This decrease is directly related to the estrogen content of the OCs (Stadel, 1986).

Neoplastic Diseases

The forms of neoplasia that are of greatest concern with the potential effects of OC use are breast cancer, cervical cancer, endometrial cancer, and ovarian cancer. There are two main reasons for the concern. First, these cancers are major causes of morbidity and mortality, particularly breast cancer in developed countries and cervical cancer in some developing countries.[1] Second, the breast, the uterus, and the ovaries are endocrine-dependent organs, and a large body of research shows that hormonally related factors, such as age at menarche and age at first birth, affect the risk of developing neoplastic diseases. Thus, any factor that alters hormones requires careful scrutiny as a possible carcinogen or anticarcinogen for these organs. In addition, cervical cancer is caused by the human papiloma virus, and contraception may modify transmission.

Complex methodological problems make the study of possible relationships between OC use and these cancers difficult. Such problems include a possible long latency period and the difficulty of evaluating factors that might alter the effects of OCs, such as age at first pregnancy for breast cancer and the number of sexual partners for cervical cancer. In fact, some studies on breast and cervical cancer among OC users have found no effect on cancer risk and others have

------

[1]Approximately 6 percent of British women and 9 percent of American women develop cancer of the breast during their lives (Schlesselman et al., 1988).

suggested increases. Since breast and cervical cancer are two of the most common cancers affecting women, the debate has taken on an urgency unlike that of other health risks. Family planning programs in the least developed countries generally lack the resources to monitor and respond adequately to these cancers. For example, Papanicolaou (Pap) screening, which is routine in developed countries, is not commonly performed in many developing countries. Although OC use clearly provides protection from the development of endometrial and ovarian cancer, its effect on other malignancies is generally unclear.

The relationship between OC use and breast cancer is controversial. The Cancer and Steroid Hormone study, the largest study to date, was conducted in eight regions of the United States from 1980 to 1982 (Centers for Disease Control and National Institute of Child Health and Human Development, 1986). This study found no increased risk of breast cancer among pill users, regardless of length of use or OC formulation. Even groups known to be at high risk, such as women with prior benign breast disease or a family history of breast cancer, nulliparous women, or those who had a late age at first full-term pregnancy, were unaffected by OC use. Controversy centers on long-term OC use, use at an early age, or use before the first full-term pregnancy. One study showed a higher rate of premenopausal breast cancer among women who used "high-progestin" OCs before age 25. Another study of women with long-term OC use before the birth of their first child found the risk of breast cancer as much as doubled in some cases (Pike et al., 1983; McPherson et al., 1983; Meirek et al., 1986). Although a subsequent analysis of the CASH data that replicated the analysis made by Pike and McPherson contradicted their findings, a recent analysis of the data from the CASH study suggests that very long-term OC use may decrease the age of onset of breast cancer for a small subset of nulliparous women without an appreciable impact for women in the aggregate (Stadel et al., 1988).

Breast cancer is uncommon among women in developing countries, and premenopausal breast cancer in these populations is rare. While there may be increased risk in small, select subgroups, in the aggregate there is probably no appreciable increase in risk. McPherson et al. (1983) have suggested that any possible risk of breast cancer associated with OC use at early ages may not become apparent until at least 20 years after that use, in which case researchers may not be able to detect such a relationship at the present time. The CASH study has found no increased risk of breast cancer within 10 to 15 years after use, even when use began at early ages (Schlesselman et al., 1988). The preponderance of epidemiologic studies suggest that OCs do not increase the risk of breast cancer, and any increase that may exist for certain subgroups of women is not great. Moreover, the inconsistencies among studies suggest that there may be methodological problems in the investigation of this complex disease.

According to available data, cancer of the cervix is the most frequent malignancy among women in developing countries (Lunt, 1984). No definite causal relationship has been established between OC use and cervical cancer. Some of the major epidemiologic studies conducted have found no increased risk and some have found significantly increased risk, at least in certain subgroups (Piper, 1985; Brinton et al., 1986; Ebeling et al., 1987; Irwin et al., 1988). A large study by the World Health Organization, which included many developing countries, found some indication of increased risk with prolonged OC use (World Health Organization, 1985a), but these studies have serious methodological problems, most notably a detection bias caused by increased Pap screening of OC users compared with nonusers and differences in sexual behavior among users and nonusers of OCs (Piper, 1985; Swan and Petitti, 1982). More recent studies have attempted to address these methodological problems, but the results remain conflicting. While OCs probably do not dramatically increase the overall risk of cervical dysplasia or cancer, long-term OC use or use by specific subgroups of women may increase the risk. Two large British cohort studies have shown a higher incidence of cervical neoplasia among oral contraceptive users (Vessey et al., 1983; Beral et al., 1988). The most important conclusion from the conflict over these results is the importance of annual Pap screening in the prevention of invasive cervical cancer.

OCs have been associated with malignant melanoma (skin cancer), but the association is rather weak and possibly confounded by differences in exposure to sunlight (Stadel, 1986). Some studies do suggest an increase within certain subgroups of women, particularly those with long-term use (Bain et al., 1982; Beral et al., 1984; Holly et al., 1983; Ramcharan et al., 1981). Due to the rarity of this malignancy in developing countries, however, the attributable risk is quite low and not very important for public health policy.

Recent case-control studies have found an increased risk of hepatocellular carcinoma (liver cancer) among OC users, largely confined to long-term users (Forman et al., 1986; Neuberger et al., 1986; Henderson et al., 1983). Unfortunately, these studies all had small sample sizes and methodological problems that may have biased the results. Since hepatocellular carcinoma is extremely rare in developed countries, the attributable risk is very low. The disease is a much more common problem in many developing countries, especially where there is a high prevalence of chronic hepatitis B. The interrelationships among OC use, hepatitis B, and liver cancer are not well understood. The World Health Organization is conducting a multicenter case-control study in three developing countries to address the question.

It is clear that OC use increases the risk of hepatocellular adenoma (HCA), a rare, benign tumor of the liver that can cause serious intra-abdominal hemorrhage and death. The case fatality rate is approximately 8 percent (Rooks et al., 1979). The risk attributable to OC use is very low, estimated to be about 2 cases of HCA per 100,000 users per year among women who have used OCs five years or more (Stadel, 1986).

Other Effects

It has been suggested that OC use might accelerate the appearance of gall bladder disease in susceptible women (Royal College of General Practitioners, 1982), although evidence for this hypothesis is limited. Early studies (Boston Collaborative Drug Surveillance Program, 1974; Royal College of General Practitioners, 1982) suggested that the risk of gall bladder disease might be increased in OC users. Recent studies and further analysis of information from British studies, which had first shown an increased risk of gallbladder disease in OC users (Layde et al., 1982; Wingrave and Kay, 1982), have failed to confirm this association.

There have been extensive studies of the effects on pregnancy outcome of hormonal contraceptive use prior to or during pregnancy. Although there are some reports of adverse effects, the majority of studies show no increased risks, and several comprehensive reviews of the literature have concluded that in utero exposure to synthetic steroids at the doses used for contraception does not result in significant deleterious effects on fetal growth or development (Wilson and Brent, 1981; World Health Organization, 1981; Simpson, 1985).

Even at low doses, the estrogen component of combination OCs has been shown to suppress milk volume in lactating mothers. Progestin-only contraceptives, including the minipill and long-acting methods discussed below, do not suppress milk production and can be used by breastfeeding women (World Health Organization, 1981). Although the synthetic hormones of the pill do pass on to the suckling infant, no adverse effects have been observed. Some reports have postulated an association between birth defects and the use of hormonal contraceptives prior to or during pregnancy. However, the majority of studies show no increased risks of deleterious effects on fetal growth or development (Wilson and Brent, 1981; World Health Organization, 1981; Simpson, 1985).

INTRAUTERINE DEVICES

The intrauterine device (IUD), which is inserted and remains in the uterus, prevents conception through several modes of action. IUDs may be medicated or nonmedicated; examples include the inert Lippes Loop, Copper-T (medicated with copper), and Progestasert (medicated with progesterone). The IUD is highly effective, having a failure rate of less than 6 percent in the first year of use. Many failures are due to undetected IUD expulsion (Trussell and Kost, 1987). It appears that new copper IUDs have a much lower failure rate of 1 to 2 percent. Rates of IUD use vary widely among countries. Partly because of its widespread use in China, the IUD is the most commonly used, reversible method of birth control in the world. IUDs are currently used by roughly 79 million women, nearly 58 million of whom live in China (United Nations, 1989).

Because IUDs appear to prevent both intrauterine and ectopic pregnancies, the overall risk of ectopic pregnancy is decreased by IUD use by about 60 percent, according to U.S. and multinational WHO studies (Ory and the Women's Health Study, 1981; Gray, 1984). However, 5 to 15 percent of IUD-associated pregnancies are ectopic, indicating that the IUD is more effective at preventing intrauterine pregnancies. Progesterone-releasing IUDs decrease menstrual blood loss and dysmenorrhea (Hatcher et al., 1988). No other noncontraceptive health benefits to IUD use have been identified.

Major health risks that have been associated with IUD use include pelvic inflammatory disease, tubal infertility, septic abortion, spontaneous abortion, and uterine perforation. The attributable mortality risk is extremely low in the United States, estimated at 1 to 2 deaths per 100,000 users and was mainly due to the now discontinued Dalkon Shield (Ory et al., 1983). Where access to medical facilities is poor and diagnosis and treatment of complications are delayed, mortality rates may be higher.

Unlike other modern methods of temporary contraception, the IUD increases the risk of pelvic inflammatory disease (Grimes, 1987). PID is usually, although not always, the result of sexually transmitted diseases (STDs). As a result, much of the risk of PID attributed to IUD use is mainly in women who are at increased risk for developing STDs. In the United States, women using IUD types other than the Dalkon Shield have been found to have about 1.5 to 2.0 times greater risk of PID than women using no method. Corresponding data in developing countries shows a relative risk of 2.3 (Gray and Campbell, 1984). The risk is largely concentrated in the first few months after IUD insertion, because insertion may introduce bacteria into the uterus (Lee et al., 1988).

The presence of PID has been clearly linked to subsequent tubal infertility. Two U.S. case-control studies found that the risk of tubal infertility among nulliparous women who ever used an IUD was double that of nonusers (Daling et al., 1985; Cramer et al., 1985). Apparently, this increased risk of tubal infertility is related to the presence of PID, even if PID is never recognized clinically. However, women who reported having only one sexual partner had no increased risk of tubal infertility associated with IUD use (Cramer et al., 1985). Therefore, in populations in which STDs are a major problem, it may be less advisable to promote IUD use. In countries such as China, however, where STDs are uncommon, the IUD is a safe and acceptable method.

If a pregnancy does occur with an IUD in place, a spontaneous abortion is likely, occurring in 50 percent of cases in which the IUD is left in place and 25 percent of cases in which it is removed (Hatcher et al., 1988). When the IUD is left in place, septic abortion in the second trimester may result and can possibly be fatal to the IUD user.

Perforation of the uterus may occur during IUD insertion but this is relatively rare, probably occurring in less than 1 percent of insertions, and usually is not serious (Hatcher et al., 1988). The risk of perforation is substantially increased among breastfeeding women and women between weeks 1 and 8 after delivery (but less during the first 4 or 5 days postpartum), evidently due to softer uterine musculature (Heartwell and Schlesselman, 1983). In general, it is recommended that the IUD be removed when perforation occurs.

BARRIER METHODS

Because they may prevent transmission of sexually transmitted diseases, including the human immunodeficiency virus (HIV), a great deal of attention is being focused on spermicides and barrier methods of contraception, principally condoms, diaphragms, and sponges. The United Nations estimates that 48 million women or their partners use these methods, but this number may be growing rapidly (United Nations, 1989). The effectiveness of these methods is highly dependent on user motivation and compliance. As a result, average failure rates tend to be higher than for any other modern method of contraception.

Condoms are a very safe method of birth control, but their effectiveness as a contraceptive and as a disease prophylactic depends on consistent and proper use. Failure rates are estimated to be as high as 12 percent per year in practice (Trussell and Kost, 1987). A number of in vitro studies have demonstrated that latex condoms are effective barriers to herpes simplex virus type 2, chlamydia trachomatis, cytomegalovirus, and HIV. Condoms evidently reduce the transmission of organisms present in the semen, such as Neisseria gonorrhoeae, hepatitis B virus, and Trichomonas vaginalis (Conant et al., 1984; Judson et al., in press; Katznelson et al., 1984; Conant et al., 1986; Stone et al., 1986).

Data regarding in vivo condom use and STDs is limited. Several studies have found a lower frequency of gonorrhea and HIV infection among condom users and/or their partners (Barlow, 1977; Hart, 1974; Hooper et al., 1978; Fischl et al., 1987; Centers for Disease Control, 1987). However, these studies are confounded by the fact that condom users are likely to differ from nonusers in many important characteristics (Feldblum and Fortney, 1988). Still, while the evidence is inconclusive, available data suggest that condoms may be quite effective STD prophylactics (Horsburgh et al., 1987). Their failure to protect is explained more probably by misuse than by product failure (Centers for Disease Control, 1988).

Spermicides are chemical agents that inactivate sperm in the vagina before they can move into the upper genital tract. The contraceptive sponge with spermicides may provide some protection against STDs, although, as with other barrier methods, the effectiveness of this contraceptive is highly dependent on user compliance. Failure rates in the first year of use may be as high as 18 percent among nulliparous women and close to 30 percent among parous women (Trussell and Kost, 1987). Laboratory and clinical evidence suggests that their virucidal effects may inhibit the growth of Neiserria gonorrhoeae (Cowan and Cree, 1973; Singh et al., 1972), herpes simplex virus type 2 (Singh et al., 1976), and HIV (Hicks et al., 1985). Although evidence is sparse, there is some indication that spermicides also protect against cervical cancer, which has been associated with the human papilloma virus (Spring and Gruber, 1985).

The sponge also has attendant health risks. Sponge users may be at increased risk of vaginal candidiasis, because normal bacterial growth is suppressed by certain types of spermicide, which leads to the overgrowth of candida (Rosenberg et al., 1987). There is also an association between the sponge and toxic shock syndrome (TSS), which in severe cases can lead to shock, coma, or death. Sponge users are apparently at 10.5 times greater risk of TSS than women using no barrier method (Schwartz et al., 1989). However, the attributable risk is low, since TSS is an extremely rare disease.

The diaphragm (with spermicide), like the condom, if used correctly and consistently, can be an effective contraceptive. Because of inadequate motivation, improper fitting, or inconsistent use, the average failure rate is roughly 18 percent per year (Trussell and Kost, 1987). The diaphragm appears to reduce the risk of gonorrhea, PID, and tubal infertility (Jick et al., 1982; Kelaghan et al., 1982; Cramer et al., 1987). Several studies have shown cervical dysplasia and cervical neoplasia to be less common among users (Wright et al., 1978; Harris et al., 1980; Celentano et al., 1987). Since diaphragms and sponges are almost always used with spermicides, it is difficult to separate the specific effects of each.

As with the sponge, the risk of TSS is significantly increased for diaphragm users (Schwartz et al., 1989). Still, the attributable risk is only about 0.2 percent annually. A less serious, but more frequent, complication associated with diaphragm use is urinary tract infections, occurring 2 to 3 times more often among users than nonusers (Foxman and Frerichs, 1985; Fihn et al., 1985; Vessey et al., 1987).

LONG-ACTING CONTRACEPTIVES

Several long-acting contraceptive methods have been developed, consisting mainly of injectables and implants. Usage is still relatively low, with just over 6 million women estimated to be using injectables (United Nations, 1989). These methods are highly effective and convenient to use and give protection from pregnancy from one month to five years. All contain a progestin, which may lead to a disturbance of the menstrual cycle.

Injectables

Two injectable progestins, Depo-Provera (DMPA) and Noristerat (NET), have been approved in over 90 countries worldwide.[2] Estimated failure rates in the first year of use are between 0.3 and 0.4 percent, depending on the kind of progestin

---

[2] Neither DMPA nor NET has been approved for use in the United States. See Richard and Lasaghna (1987) for a review of the debate on approval.

used (Trussell and Kost, 1987). Injections are usually given every 8 to 12 weeks. Injectables prevent pregnancy by inhibiting ovulation, thickening cervical mucous, and altering the endometrial lining, which inhibits implantation (Liskin and Quillin, 1982).

The relationship between the risk of cancer and the use of injectables, particularly DMPA, remains controversial. The largest epidemiologic study yet published is an ongoing case-control study conducted by the World Health Organization. This study has found no increased risk of breast and endometrial cancer, and an analysis of invasive cervical cancer was deemed inconclusive. Final results concerning breast and cervical cancer are expected in the near future from this study and from a study in New Zealand. These and other studies have been hindered by small sample sizes and short durations of exposure. Animal data suggest that DMPA may increase the risk of breast and endometrial cancer (World Health Organization, 1986a).

Reported metabolic effects of the use of injectables include changes in blood pressure and insulin, cholesterol, and triglyceride levels (Liskin et al., 1987; WHO, 1986b). Various studies of DMPA and NET users have found both increases and decreases in total cholesterol and HDL-cholesterol. The findings are thus inconsistent and none has shown clear clinical significance (Liskin et al., 1987). No studies have been published on the possible associations between DMPA or NET use and the risk of cardiovascular disease. Unlike OCs, injectables appear to have little effect on the coagulation and fibrinolytic systems that affect blood clotting.

Amenorrhea or irregular, unpredictable bleeding episodes are the most commonly reported problems with injectables and the primary reason for terminating use (World Health Organization, 1978; Swenson et al., 1980; World Health Organization, 1987b). One-half to two-thirds of users have no regular menstrual cycles in the first year of use (Liskin et al., 1987). After one year of use, as many as 50 percent of users will be amenorrheac. The occurrence of heavy bleeding is rare, occurring in 0.5 percent of users. Conversely, since bleeding is often lighter than normal, increased hemoglobin levels have been reported (World Health Organization, 1986b).

Injectables appear to have no permanent effect on fertility, although ovulation may be inhibited for four to nine months or more after the last injection (Liskin et al., 1987; Pardthaisong et al., 1980; Affandi et al., 1987). Injectables may protect against PID by causing changes in the cervical mucus (Gray, 1985).

Injectable progestins may protect against endometrial and ovarian cancers. A WHO case-control study found a reduced risk of endometrial cancer in DMPA users, but the sample was quite small and results are inconclusive (World Health Organization, 1986a). There are even fewer data regarding ovarian cancer. However, since injectables prevent ovulation, as do OCs, it is hypothesized that injectables will also decrease the incidence of ovarian cancer; preliminary results from the WHO study support this possibility.

Implants

The Norplant subdermal implant system is another highly effective progestational contraceptive. One-inch-long plastic rods are surgically implanted under the skin of the upper arm and are left in place for several years. The progestin levonorgestrel is slowly released and remains effective for three to five years. The implants have a cumulative five-year net pregnancy rate of less than 2 percent in most studies (Segal, 1988).

Like injectables, the most common side effect of implants is disturbance of the menstrual cycle. Episodes of abnormal bleeding diminish with duration of use but, unlike injectables, the implants can be removed if there are extreme complications. Norplant users are generally protected from ectopic pregnancy since ovulation is suppressed. Transient ovarian cysts occur in a small percentage of women using Norplant, although the cysts eventually regress (Salah et al., 1987; Diaz et al., 1987). Permanent infertility appears not to be a problem (Sivin et al., 1983; Diaz et al., 1987; Affandi et al., 1987). Several studies have shown that fecundity quickly returns after the implants are removed. No changes have been found in liver function, carbohydrate metabolism, blood coagulation, blood pressure, or body weight (Liskin et al., 1987). Of particular importance in the use of implants is the very low blood level of progestogen, which is much lower than with other steroid contraceptives.

STERILIZATION

Sterilization is the most widely used contraceptive method in the world. More than 108 million women and 41 million men have undergone sterilization procedures (United Nations, 1989). Sterilization is safe and highly effective; most of the health risks are associated with poor anesthetic or surgical technique.

Pregnancy identified after tubal sterilization may result from conception before sterilization or from unsuccessful sterilization. Failure rates, which vary by method of tubal occlusion, surgical expertise, and patient characteristics, are overall estimated to be between 2 and 4 per 1,000 in the first year of use (Trussell and Kost, 1987). When female sterilization failure occurs, ectopic gestation is more likely than intrauterine gestation, but the absolute likelihood of ectopic pregnancy is actually lower than that associated with use of no method or even IUDs.

Tubal sterilization is usually performed via an abdominal incision. A vaginal approach offers the advantage of producing no visible scar, but such a procedure increases the risk of pelvic infection and thus is used less frequently. The fallopian tubes may be blocked by tying (with or without removal), by coagulation, using unipolar or bipolar current, or by mechanical occlusion with silastic bands or clips. All procedures except conventional laparotomy can be safely performed using local anesthesia, thus avoiding the hazards inherent in the use of general anesthesia.

Studies suggest that tubal sterilization is a remarkably safe surgical procedure. The case-fatality rate has been reported as low as 4 per 100,000 procedures in U.S. hospitals (Peterson et al., 1982) but as high as 19 per 100,000 procedures in Bangladesh (Grimes et al., 1982). Most deaths are caused by complications related to use of anesthesia, even when general anesthesia is not used. Deaths have occurred from hemorrhage and thermal injury as well (Peterson et al., 1983). Reports regarding nonfatal complications vary. In general, such studies indicate that major morbidity is uncommon and varies by surgical approach, anesthetic technique, and tubal occlusion method.

No important long-term negative physiological effects of tubal sterilization have been reported in the literature. Much concern has focused on menstrual abnormalities, the so-called post-tubal syndrome, which was identified by a number of studies prior to 1980. These early studies had methodological problems; better designed, more recent studies have found no evidence of a post-tubal syndrome. When menstrual changes did occur, about as many women experienced improvement in symptoms as experienced a deleterious change (Bhiwandiwala et al., 1983). Many of the observed changes were attributable to cessation of OC or IUD use. Studies have found conflicting results on the question of an increased risk of hysterectomy following sterilization. It has been postulated that any observed correlation may be explained by the fact that, once a woman has been sterilized, either she or her physician may more quickly resort to surgical management of any gynecologic problem.

Male sterilization, or vasectomy, is the cutting or occluding of the vas deferens to prevent sperm transport. Although safe, simple, and highly effective, vasectomy is not popular in most countries. Most users reside in the United States, the United Kingdom, China, and India. Access to services and motivational factors have been cited as reasons for the generally low level of use. Few studies report any pregnancies after vasectomies and, of those that do, most have reported failure rates below 1 percent, with most failures attributable to unprotected intercourse shortly after vasectomy or spontaneous rejoining of the vas (Trussell and Kost, 1987).

The procedure consists of isolating the vas deferens, then occluding it by ligation (the most common approach), coagulation, or clip application. Local anesthesia without premedication is most often used. The risk of death attributable to vasectomy is extremely low. The Association for Voluntary Surgical Contraception has recorded only two vasectomy-related deaths associated with over 160,000 procedures in programs it supported (Ross et al., 1985).

Research has consistently failed to identify long-term health risks attributable to vasectomy. In contrast to animal findings, at least six epidemiologic studies in humans, including a large study in China, have indicated that the risk of myocardial infarction is not increased in the 10 years following vasectomy (Goldacre et al., 1978, 1979; Walker et al., 1981; Petitti et al., 1982; Massey et al., 1984; Perrin et al., 1984). Possible relationships between vasectomy and prostatic disease have been examined (Sidney, 1987; Ross et al., 1985). With the exception of one recent study (Honda et al., 1988), no association between vasectomy and prostatic disease has been found, and a plausible alternative explanation for the results was made by the authors of that study. Still controversial is the relationship between vasectomy and subsequent genito-urinary tract diseases, such as kidney stones (urolithiasis). One recent report has found a 70 percent increased risk of kidney stones among men who had undergone vasectomy (Kronmal et al., 1988). Other studies have found no relationship, but the possibility warrants further evaluation.

TRADITIONAL METHODS

Traditional methods of contraception include periodic abstinence or rhythm, withdrawal, douche, or complete abstinence. Unsupplemented breastfeeding on demand postpones the onset of ovulation and may thus also be considered a form of contraception. It is difficult to measure the use of these methods, since they may be practiced without being called contraception. The United Nations reports that over 77 million women rely on one of these methods (United Nations, 1989). Periodic abstinence and withdrawal are much less effective than most of the modern methods already discussed, with failure rates around 15-20 percent in the first year of use (Trussell and Kost, 1987).

That breastfeeding can provide considerable protection against pregnancy is well documented (see Hatcher et al., 1988, for a review). Pregnancy rates in populations depend on breastfeeding prevalence and practices. Hatcher et al. (1988:117) conclude: "Breastfeeding can be an effective method of fertility control for a population, but breastfeeding effectiveness is unpredictable for the individual woman, particularly with western patterns of breastfeeding and supplementation."

Periodic abstinence or rhythm is based on awareness of variation in the woman's fecundity over the menstrual cycle using the calendar, basal body temperature, and/or the character of cervical mucus. Rhythm has no health risks or noncontraceptive benefits for a woman. There may be an increased risk that an old, rather than a fresh, egg will be fertilized, possibly leading to a higher risk of fetal wastage or birth defects. Animal studies have shown that aged gametes may be associated with increased early abortions and increased birth defects, and equivocal, limited data suggest an increase in spontaneous abortions. But studies on humans have been unconvincing, either to support or discount the possible effects (Hatcher et al., 1988; Kambic et al., 1988).

It is uncertain how frequently coitus interruptus (withdrawal) is used worldwide. There are no known biological side effects. Douching and other means of cleaning out the vagina after intercourse have been used to prevent conception ever since it was understood that ejaculation into the vagina caused pregnancy. Not only is the method highly ineffective for contraception, but it also greatly increases the risk of vaginal infection. Douching has been associated with an increased risk of PID, although the relationship may not be causal. A case-control study found that women who douched frequently had 4.4 times the risk of ectopic pregnancy (Chow et al., 1985).

DIMENSIONS OF NEW RESEARCH

Clearly, no modern method of contraception is completely free of health consequences, whether adverse or beneficial or both. Oral contraceptives, which increase the risk of a variety of cardiovascular problems, also protect against PID, ectopic pregnancy, and two cancers of the reproductive system. Barrier methods of contraception, which may reduce the transmission of sexually transmitted diseases, are also associated with an increased risk of pregnancy. Sterilization, while generally an extremely safe procedure, can be dangerous if improperly performed.

Priorities for further safety studies should be determined by the incidence of serious disease in a country. For example, where liver cancer is already problematic, contraceptive research should focus on the impact of contraceptive methods on this disease. At the same time, research must respond to case reports that are particularly unusual. A finding that 9 out of 10 cases of a rare disease were all using the same method of contraception would indicate the need for further study. These decisions are far from simple. The pervasive concerns and worries of a population or a government cannot be ignored, even when empirical data negate their importance. Still, we are left with a number of questions. At what level of incidence does an epidemiologic study become necessary? What level of risk is acceptable for the continued marketing of a specific method? How important are discomforting but nonfatal side effects?

Ongoing research to test new variations of existing contraceptive methods as well as the development of new methods must be continued. The long-term effects of most methods can be determined only after many years of use, a situation that mandates repeated and protracted study. Cohort studies are needed to evaluate the overall pattern of mortality and morbidity related to contraceptive use, and case-control studies are needed to evaluate the contraceptive-related risks for specific diseases. Moreover, ongoing surveillance of the use of all hormonal contraceptives in both developed and developing countries is crucial.

By way of conclusion, it is appropriate to put the various risks of contraceptive use into perspective. Due to the uncertainty associated with the various health risks for each method of contraception and the methodological complexities inherent in such analyses, no definitive overall risk can be calculated by method (see Ory et al., 1983, for estimates of risks). However, in developing countries, where maternal mortality is high, and diseases associated with contraception such as myocardial infarction are uncommon, there is no questions that contraception is safer than pregnancy and childbirth.

Any decision regarding contraceptive use must be based not only on the noncontraceptive risks and benefits, but also on the efficacy of the method. Each individual's life situation and the level of risk particular to his or her characteristics must be considered as well. Finally, the life consequences of childbearing for the mother and child must also be considered. We now turn to the health consequences of controlled fertility for children, again with special consideration of high-risk categories.

5

Reproductive Patterns and Children's Health

Despite the major improvements in child health that have occurred since World War II, infant and child mortality rates in many developing countries remain very high. During 1980-1985, almost 90 out of every 1,000 infants born in the developing world died before their first birthday. In contrast, there were an estimated 16 infant deaths per 1,000 births in the developed world (United Nations, 1988b). Other indicators of poor child health, such as the incidence of infectious disease and malnutrition, also remain high in many developing countries, particularly in the poorer countries in sub-Saharan Africa and South Asia.

The major difference in child health between developing and industrialized countries is that infectious and parasitic diseases, including diarrheal diseases, and malnutrition, are considerably more common in the Third World. In addition, children in developing countries are likely to have multiple conditions that increase the potential severity of illness and raise the probability of death. To illustrate differences in the distribution of causes of death in countries with different patterns of mortality, Table 5.1 shows the distributions of cause of death for infants in a high-mortality population (Recife, Brazil, in the late 1960s), a moderate-mortality population (Paraguay in 1983), and a low-mortality population (the United States in 1983). Infectious, parasitic, and respiratory diseases, like measles and diarrheal disease, account for almost two-thirds of the infant deaths in Recife, but only 6 percent of the infant deaths in the United States. Because deaths due to infectious diseases become much less common as mortality declines, congenital anomalies and conditions associated with birth and the immediate postbirth period are relatively more prominent in low-mortality populations.

TABLE 5.1   Cause of Death (Percentage of All Infant Deaths) and Infant Mortality Rate for Three Populations

Cause of Death	Recife, Brazil 1968-1981[a] High Mortality	Paraguay 1983 Moderate Mortality	United States 1983 Low Mortality
Infectious and parasitic diseases	51	23	2
Diseases of respiratory system	11	14	4
Congenital anomalies	4	4	21
Certain perinatal conditions	26	24	47
Ill-defined	8	21	14
All other		13	11
Infant mortality rate	91	51	11

[a] "Basic causes" only, by ICDD-8 Classification (from Inter-American Investigation of Mortality in Childhood).

Sources: Puffer and Serrano (1973); World Health Organization (1987a).

Causes of poor health and mortality also change during the course of childhood. Congenital problems, low birthweight, and difficulties during pregnancy or birth are more likely to affect morbidity and mortality during the neonatal period (the first month of life) than later in infancy. Certain infections, such as neonatal tetanus, are also particularly prevalent during the first month, and other infectious diseases, such as pneumonia, are significant neonatal health risks. Mortality and illness after the neonatal period, which are usually associated with infectious or parasitic diseases and poor nutrition, are more directly influenced by the environment in which a child lives than mortality and illness during the first month of life.

Specific infectious and parasitic diseases often affect children of particular ages. For example, Foster (1984) reports differential effects of measles by age, with highest mortality under age 1 and decreasing mortality thereafter. The age pattern of childhood illness in high-mortality countries often depends on breastfeeding and weaning practices. Once weaning begins, children lose the immunities provided by breast milk, and they begin to consume food that may be contaminated. After weaning, children become dependent on the family food supply, which may be inadequate, contaminated, or inappropriate for their needs. In addition, protection from maternal antibodies declines with age. Because the etiology of poor health and mortality can change considerably during infancy and childhood, it is important to consider the effect of reproductive patterns on child health separately for children of different age groups.

Previous research suggests that the risk of mortality and poor health are higher for children who are born to mothers with particular reproductive histories. Results of bivariate studies[1] usually show that infant and child mortality rates are higher for those who are:

- the firstborn, born to a young mother, or a combination;
- a higher-order birth, born to an older mother, or a combination;
- born into a family with a large final number of children ever born;
- born before or after a short interbirth interval.

It has also been hypothesized that:

- children born as a result of unwanted pregnancies are likely to be in poorer health compared with children born as a result of other pregnancies.

In this chapter we first review sources of data and analytical issues and then examine studies on the relationships between reproductive patterns and infant and child health. These studies are summarized at the end of the chapter in Appendix Table 5.A.

SOURCES OF EVIDENCE

Much of the earliest evidence linking child health and survival, particularly during infancy, with maternal age, birth order, and the timing and spacing of births was based on data from industrialized countries. Many of these studies dealt with small, select populations and had few, if any, controls for confounding factors. Recently, a number of population-based studies using more sophisticated statistical procedures and data from developing countries have provided substantially more information about these complex relationships between reproduction and health in Third World settings. Most of these studies focus on infant and child mortality as measures of health, because data on other indices of health are not as commonly available. For this reason, the results described in this chapter draw primarily on studies of the associations between reproductive patterns and child survival. Whenever possible, however, the discussion is supplemented with other information about child health, such as birthweight and illness.

Much of the recent evidence on the association between reproductive patterns and child health in developing countries comes from the World Fertility Survey

---

[1]See, for example, Rutstein (1983) for evidence on the first four types of characteristics listed.

(WFS), which were conducted between 1974 and 1982 in a number of developing countries. In these surveys, nationally representative samples of women of reproductive age were interviewed about their birth or pregnancy histories and the fate of each of their live-born children. In analyses of these data, this birth history information has been used to determine the length of the intervals preceding and following the birth of a given child, the child's birth order among his siblings, and his mother's age at the time he or she was born.

Recent analyses of data from the WFS and other retrospective survey data have demonstrated that child survival is strongly associated with longer intervals between births. This association has been found in a large number of populations with very different levels of mortality, fertility, and economic development. These studies have also shown that maternal age and birth order are significantly related to child survival in many populations. However, there are several potential problems with drawing inferences about causal relationships from analyses of these data. First, reporting errors common to retrospective fertility histories may exaggerate the relationships observed between birth spacing and child survival.[2] Second, most of the surveys contain only limited information on breastfeeding, length of gestation, birthweight, and other biomedical characteristics of the mother and child that may be important factors in the relationship between child health and reproductive patterns. Third, many of the surveys collected only limited information on socioeconomic status and other family characteristics, which may independently affect both fertility and children's health. Fourth, data imputation procedures used in the WFS may alter estimates of effects (Trussell and Rodriguez, 1989).

Because of these limitations on analyses of retrospective survey data, we also draw on the results of studies based on two other types of information. One source is a small number of studies based on data collected longitudinally in developing countries. Carefully collected longitudinal data do not suffer from the same type of systematic misreporting that affects retrospective surveys. Furthermore, longitudinal studies frequently also collect detailed data on biomedical and behavioral factors, such as length of gestation and birthweight, which may not be available in retrospective data. Unfortunately, longitudinal data have been collected in only a few populations, and, in some cases, more extensive analyses of extant data needs to be undertaken.

Another source of evidence is studies of historical populations in Europe and the United States that experienced mortality rates at the same or higher levels as those found in contemporary populations in the Third World. One advantage of historical data is that, like longitudinal data, they are less subject to the type of misreporting problems sometimes found in retrospective survey data. Historical

---

[2] Previous research has shown that respondents are more likely to omit both the birth and death of children no longer alive at the time of the interview. The women who do omit reports of children who have died will appear to have both longer birth intervals and their children will have lower mortality rates (Potter, 1988; Cleland and Sathar, 1984).

data sets, however, suffer from different types of data quality problems, including omission of events due to immigration and lapses in recordkeeping (Lynch, 1987; Bean et al., 1987). With historical data, reproductive and mortality histories cover the entire reproductive span. Comparison of results from high-mortality historical populations with those from contemporary developing countries also allows us to make inferences about whether the hypothesized relationships are common to high-mortality populations in a variety of cultural, social, and economic contexts.

Assessment of the association between reproductive variables and child survival is complicated by a number of methodological, statistical, and theoretical problems (see Potter, 1988; Rosenzweig and Schultz, 1983; Hobcraft et al., 1985; Hobcraft, 1987; Pebley and Millman, 1986). First, the reproductive variables of interest are likely to be highly correlated. For example, higher child mortality observed among children born to teenage mothers may actually be a consequence of the fact that a large proportion of these births are first births. Unless both variables are included simultaneously in the analysis, higher risks of mortality may be incorrectly attributed to either one variable or the other.

Second, reverse or spurious causality complicates the interpretation of results unless adequate statistical controls are introduced for factors such as breastfeeding and the survival status of the preceding birth. For example, an apparent association between a child's mortality risk and the length of the subsequent birth interval could be due to either the child's death ending breastfeeding and leading to earlier conception of the next child, or to early weaning or no breastfeeding, which itself places the child at greater risk.

Third, certain characteristics of the family may increase the likelihood both that children in that family will be in good health and that births will be widely spaced, or that there will be a small number of children in the family. For example, women who have completed elementary education may be both more likely to use contraception to space or limit their births and to be able to provide better care for their children. In addition, in a noncontraceptive population, women who lose children will have more total births because of shorter birth intervals caused by interrupted lactation. If adequate attention is not paid to the role of unobserved heterogeneity in the design of the analysis, reproductive variables will appear to be correlated with child health, when in fact the relationship is not causal.[3] Because fertility and child health are both affected by parental choices, unobserved variables—environmental constraints, biologically fixed characteristics, or parent preferences—can affect both outcomes, and any association between fertility and child health may be a biased estimate of the causal relationship. There is no consensus about the most appropriate way to eliminate potential bias.

---

[3] This problem can also be viewed as simultaneous-equations bias, the consequences of which are well described in the economics literature (see, for example, Schultz, 1984).

Many recent studies of reproductive patterns and child health have used multivariate statistical methods in an attempt to control for some of these problems. Although limitations remain in the studies on which our assessment is based, we rely principally on analyses that employed multivariate methods and introduced statistical controls for potentially confounding factors. Both the theoretical models and statistical methods used in this research continue to evolve.

EFFECTS OF BEING FIRSTBORN AND YOUNG MATERNAL AGE

Children born to teenage mothers and children who are firstborn are generally at higher risk of dying than children born to mothers in their twenties and children of birth order 2, 3, and 4. In several studies, both young maternal age and first birth order remained important predictors of infant and child mortality, even when the other variable is held constant. These results indicate that the estimated effect of young maternal age is not due solely to the fact that births to young mothers are more likely to be first births, nor is the estimated effect of being firstborn due solely to the fact of being more likely to have a young mother.

First Births

The available evidence from many countries suggests that the negative effects of being firstborn may be limited to the first year of life. In an analysis of World Fertility Survey data from 34 countries, Hobcraft (1987) found that the average estimated risk of dying across all countries for firstborn children compared with children of birth order 2 and 3 with optimal spacing was 1.7 for the neonatal period, 1.5 for the postneonatal period. No excessive risk was found for the toddler period (ages 1 to 2) and for childhood (ages 2 to 5).[4] It is important to note, however, that there is considerable variation in the size of the relative risks for first births among the national populations included in the Hobcraft analysis and among the populations of other studies that have looked at the same issue. Indeed, in five countries in the Hobcraft analysis, firstborn children do not experience higher risks of death. The results from other multivariate analyses are mixed: some find higher risks for first births and others do not. We have examined variations in the sizes of the relative risks for first births across countries and found no systematic relationship between the relative risks and either total fertility rates or infant mortality rates.

---

[4] The figures given in the text are the relative odds of dying for firstborn children compared with children who were of second or third births with favorable birth spacing (more than 24 months) and with no prior child deaths. Hobcraft (1987) points out that the effects of being a first birth may be somewhat exaggerated by comparison only with second and third births, when there were no previous child deaths (see Hobcraft, 1987, pg. 8, for further discussion).

Hypotheses about the higher risks of mortality and poor health associated with first births usually center around physiological adjustment of the mother to her first pregnancy. There is considerable evidence to indicate that first pregnancies and births have a higher rate of complications than subsequent pregnancies. For example, Fortney et al. (1985) present evidence from 86 hospitals, mostly in developing countries, indicating that, although the incidence of complications of delivery, such as breech presentation, is not higher for first births, perinatal mortality rates associated with such complicated deliveries of first births are higher. Other complications of pregnancy, such as pregnancy-induced hypertension, appear to be more common for women who are pregnant for the first time (Haaga, 1989). These complications of pregnancy and childbirth result in both a higher incidence of maternal morbidity and mortality and in a greater risk of morbidity and mortality for infants.

There is also evidence that the incidence of low birthweight (less than 2,500 g) is higher among first births (DaVanzo et al., 1984; Niswander and Gordon, 1972). Recent reviews by Haaga (1989) and Kramer (1987) suggest that much of this higher incidence of low birthweight among firstborn children is due to intrauterine growth retardation rather than to prematurity.

Haaga (1989) suggests that the higher incidence of malaria infestation in some areas may account for some of the excess health risk to firstborn children during first pregnancies. The presence of malarial parasites in the placenta is associated with low birthweight. Research in sub-Saharan Africa indicates that women having their first pregnancy have twice the rate of placental malaria as women who have already been pregnant before (Bray and Anderson, 1979; McGregor et al., 1983). However, more evidence is needed before we can assess the role of malaria in differences in infant mortality rates by birth order.

Young Maternal Age

The Hobcraft (1987) cross-sectional analysis of WFS data indicates that the risks for children of teenagers are higher than for those of older women. On average, across 34 countries, Hobcraft found that the odds of dying for the children of teenage mothers were 1.2 times those for mothers ages 25 to 34 during the neonatal period, 1.4 times during the postneonatal period, 1.6 times during the toddler years, and 1.3 times during childhood years. Again, however, there was substantial variation among countries included in the study in terms of the size of the effects of young maternal age.

At least two explanations for the observed association between young maternal age and elevated risks of child mortality have been suggested. First, pregnancies that occur before full maternal growth or physical maturation is achieved may place both the woman and her child at greater risk of complications of pregnancy and childbirth. There is some evidence that very young maternal age may have negative consequences for children because of the greater likelihood of birth trauma (Aitken and Walls, 1986), but Haaga concludes that the evidence that competition for nutrients exists between maternal growth and fetal growth in women who have not yet reached full physical maturity is weak. To study the biological mechanisms involved in the relationship between young maternal age and child health ideally requires analyses that look at the effects of gynecological age (the stage of physical maturation that a girl has achieved), rather than chronological age. This issue may be more salient in developing countries in which the mean age at menarche is relatively late (Foster et al., 1986) and, in some countries, the proportion of girls having their first birth shortly after menarche is considerably higher. Because of the difficulty of assessing gynecological or biological age for large samples, studies on which our conclusions are based rely principally on chronological age. Even if we are limited to chronological age, it is important to distinguish between very young maternal ages (less than 17), which may be particularly problematic, and the later teenage years (18-19), which may be optimal, at least physiologically, for childbearing. However, most of the research related to maternal age considers all ages less than 20 together.

The second possible explanation is that young women who become pregnant are less likely to receive early and adequate prenatal care, more likely to be from poor families, and less able to care for their children because they have not reached full psychological maturity themselves. Recent reviews of evidence linking teenage childbearing to poor child health in the United States (Strobino, 1987; Geronimus, 1987; McAnarney, 1987) have concluded that the main reason for this association is that teenage mothers are more likely to be socially disadvantaged than women who give birth at older ages. This explanation is probably less applicable in many developing countries, in which births to teenagers are more common and usually take place within marriage or a socially sanctioned union. Furthermore, evidence from several studies in developing countries suggests that the association between higher risks of child mortality and young maternal age persists even when socioeconomic status is held constant. However, it may be that the measures of socioeconomic status and living conditions used in these studies do not adequately capture characteristics common to teenage mothers in developing countries that affect child survival, such as inadequate use of prenatal care.

Summary

From the evidence available, we conclude that firstborn children and children born to very young mothers are at greater-than-average risk of mortality and poor health. In the case of firstborn children, there is some evidence to suggest that there are physiological reasons for this greater risk. In particular, women who are pregnant for the first time are more likely to experience complications of pregnancy and childbirth, their babies are more likely to be of low birthweight, and, in some areas, maternal malaria, which is more common during first pregnancies, may contribute to the higher mortality of firstborn children.

The issue of age is more complicated. Although some evidence suggests that births to very young girls may be at higher risk for physiological reasons, the effect may be principally social and psychological for older teenagers. Even in countries with relatively high birth rates for girls younger than 17, the proportion of all teenage births that occur to very young teenagers (17 and younger) is relatively small. The evidence from studies that group teenagers of all ages together is mixed. More research is needed in this area.

EFFECTS OF HIGH BIRTH ORDER AND OLDER MATERNAL AGE

The available evidence suggests that the detrimental effects of high birth order and older maternal age on child survival are not as important as the effects of young maternal age, being firstborn, or close spacing between births. Results of multivariate studies of this issue have produced divergent results. Hobcraft et al. (1985) conclude that much of the elevated risk attributed to older maternal ages and higher birth orders is probably produced by close birth spacing. Although their results vary considerably among the 34 countries studied, on average the risk was higher for parities 7 and higher. Pebley and Stupp (1987) also report higher risks for children of older mothers and higher birth orders in Guatemala, but neither Gubhaju (1986) nor DaVanzo et al. (1983) find significant effects of older maternal age and high birth order on child survival in Nepal and Peninsular Malaysia, respectively. Two studies using historical data (Bean et al., 1987, and Knodel and Hermalin, 1984) did find higher infant mortality at older maternal ages and higher birth orders. However, Knodel and Hermalin show that final sibship size (i.e., the total number of births the mother eventually has) is a more important correlate than birth order, and Bean et al. found that the likelihood that all previous children survived through infancy was more important for survival than birth order for second- and higher-order births.

There is less evidence concerning independent effects of older maternal age on infant health than there is on birth order. Older maternal age is associated with an increased incidence of congenital abnormalities, including Down's syndrome (Hansen, 1986; Hook, 1985), but these congenital abnormalities are a relatively minor cause of infant death in developing countries (Haaga, 1989).

EFFECTS OF SHORT BIRTH INTERVALS

The evidence concerning the effects of birth spacing on child survival and health is more consistent than that concerning the effects of high parity and maternal age. Studies based on very different types of data from culturally and socially diverse populations consistently find a negative association between short birth intervals and a child's chances of survival. This is especially true for the length of the previous interval, i.e., the length of time since the birth of the previous child.

Results from several studies indicate that the crucial period is up to 24 months after the birth of the previous child. Children born within this period are at considerably higher risk than children born after longer previous birth intervals. For example, the results from the Hobcraft (1987) study show the average risk of dying for children born within two years of a previous sibling relative to children born after longer intervals is approximately 1.8 in the first year and 1.3 for toddlers (ages 1 to 2) and in the childhood years (ages 2 to 5). Most studies have found that the mortality risks associated with short intervals are significantly higher when the child who begins the interval dies before the next child is born. This may be due to household or familial effects that increase risk for all children. However, these studies did not control for potentially confounding factors, such as breastfeeding, that may also influence the relationship.

There is considerably less evidence on the association between length of previous birth interval and other health indices such as birthweight and growth. Low birthweight may be due to intrauterine growth retardation, defined as birthweight less than the 10th percentile for gestational age, or preterm delivery, defined as gestational age less than 37 weeks.[5] Studies of the relationship between birth interval length and birthweight are complicated by the fact that preterm births, by their nature, have shorter periods of gestation and thus shorter birth intervals. These confounding effects associated with preterm births need to be controlled to estimate the association between birth interval length and birthweights accurately.

Although the risk of death is increased for all low-birthweight infants, the risk is highest for preterm babies, especially those with very low birthweights. Both differentiation between intrauterine growth retardation and preterm births and measurement of birth-to-conception intervals are necessary to determine accurately possible relationships. Ferraz et al. (1988) report a significantly increased relative risk of intrauterine growth retardation associated with interpregnancy intervals of six months or less. No association was found between birth-to-conception intervals and preterm delivery. Several investigations have shown an association between short intervals between the birth of a child and the conception of the following child and an increased risk of low birthweight, though this was not observed in studies in Norway and the United States (Erickson and Bjerkedal, 1978; Klebanoff, 1988).

Fewer studies have attempted to investigate the association between child survival and the length of the following interval. Excess mortality of those born before a short succeeding interval may be due to early cessation of breastfeeding and resultant inadequate feeding and increased exposure to pathogens at vulnerable ages, but estimation of such effects must also allow for reverse causation.

---

[5] Kramer (1987) examined the extensive literature on low birthweight, concluding that research findings are frequently conflicting because of a failure to distinguish between intrauterine growth retardation and prematurity, inadequate control for confounding variables, and lack of statistical power.

The death of the child may itself cause the subsequent interval to be short either through a biological effect (abrupt end of lactation leading to short postpartum amenorrhea) or a behavioral effect (parents trying to replace the lost child quickly). Nonetheless, studies that have examined the issue and controlled for reverse causality have generally found that short subsequent intervals are associated with higher mortality risks for the child whose birth begins the interval. For example, on the average across 34 countries, Hobcraft (1987) found that the risk of dying as a toddler (i.e., in the second year of life) for children whose mother had another birth within 12 months of their own was 2.2 times the risk of children whose mothers delayed the next birth for at least 18 months. As in the case of other results cited above, it is important to note that the risks associated with being born before a very short interval vary considerably among the countries included in the Hobcraft study and in other studies that have examined this relationship.

Possible Factors

There are several mechanisms through which short birth spacing may increase a child's risk of dying. Although some evidence is available concerning some of these mechanisms, the information is not sufficient to allow us to say with confidence exactly why close birth spacing is associated with higher child mortality. Furthermore, the relative importance of each mechanism may vary considerably among populations.

One mechanism through which closely spaced births may affect a child's health is by reducing the time available to the mother to recover from one pregnancy before beginning the next, leading to the birth of a less-than- normally healthy child. Breastfeeding and, to a lesser extent, pregnancy are significant drains on a woman's nutritional resources (Merchant and Martorell, 1988). There is evidence that short birth and pregnancy intervals are associated with low birthweight (Fedrick and Adelstein, 1973; DaVanzo et al., 1984; Fortney and Higgins, 1984). However, several studies that have attempted to link indices of maternal health to short birth spacing have not produced persuasive evidence that so-called maternal depletion accounts for the association between birth spacing and child survival except in extremely malnourished populations (Winikoff and Sullivan, 1987; Ferraz et al., 1988; Costello, 1986; Pebley and DaVanzo, 1988).

A second possible mechanism is that in families with closely spaced births, there may be greater competition among children of approximately the same age for scarce family resources. These resources may include not only food, clothing, and living space but also parental time and attention. Competition between siblings may occur because of either short previous or subsequent intervals.

One obvious example of competition occurring because of a short subsequent interval is that the conception of another child often means that the mother weans the child she is breastfeeding. Analyses of the determinants of infant and child mortality that have investigated the effects of breastfeeding have routinely shown that breastfeeding is a very important correlate of child survival in developing countries. Thus, it is appears that one of the reasons for the observed relationship between short subsequent interval length and higher risks of dying is earlier termination of breastfeeding. However, even when controls are introduced for breastfeeding length, a significant relationship often remains between subsequent interval length and child survival, suggesting that termination of breastfeeding does not entirely explain the association (Palloni and Millman, 1986; Cleland and Sathar, 1984; Pebley and Stupp, 1987). There is relatively little evidence available on other types of competition among closely spaced children for scarce family resources. Studies that have looked at the issue often produce contradictory results (see for example Palloni, 1985, Clark, 1981, and DaVanzo et al., 1983). This is clearly an area in which more research is needed.

A third hypothesis is that close birth spacing is associated with higher child mortality because infectious diseases may be more readily spread among siblings of similar ages who are in close physical proximity most of the time. Repeated exposure to some infectious disease organisms, which is more likely in crowded households, households with numerous children, and especially households with children of similar ages, increases both a child's risk of contracting the infection and the severity of the infection among children who do become ill (Aaby et al., 1984).

Finally, despite attempts to control for confounding factors in recent multivariate analyses, part of the observed relationship may result from spurious associations or unobserved heterogeneity, making it appear that close spacing increases the risks of poor child health. One hypothesis about the association between very short previous interbirth intervals and poor child survival is that pregnancies of shorter gestation are more likely to be associated with short previous birth intervals than full-term pregnancies, and these pregnancies of shorter gestation are more likely to result in the birth of babies who are at greater risk of dying. While this classification problem may account for part of the association between very short previous birth intervals and poorer child survival chances, the indirect evidence suggests that, in developing countries, the difference in gestational length is not the primary reason for the observed relationship. However, the dramatically higher risk of mortality associated with very short intervals may be due to gestational length (Miller, 1989; Wolfers and Scrimshaw, 1975; Pebley and Stupp, 1987).

A potentially more serious problem is that women who have shorter birth intervals may be different from other women in ways that are related to their ability to improve their children's chances for survival and good health (Rosenzweig and Schultz, 1983; Potter, 1988; Pebley and Stupp, 1987). A number of studies have attempted to take this possibility into account by controlling for social and economic characteristics of children's families. Nevertheless, some of the family characteristics that are likely to be most important in determining birth spacing and child health have not been included in these analyses.

Some characteristics of families that may affect the observed relationship are, in practice, unobservable themselves. Two examples are fecundity, or the ability to become pregnant, and frailty, or the underlying (possible genetic) predisposition toward illness; unobserved heterogeneity of this sort can be dealt with only by the use of experimental designs. Other characteristics include a family's propensity to use health and family planning services and its attitudes and the skills of its members related to planning and intervention in natural processes that are likely to be positively associated with birth spacing in developing countries. In this case, the omission of a variable for "use of health care" in an analysis explaining child health could result in overestimating the benefit of longer birth spacing.

Summary

The available evidence to date suggests that there is an important relationship between close birth spacing and poor child health. This association has been observed in a large number of diverse populations, both in developing countries and in high-mortality historical populations as well as in contemporary industrialized countries (Miller, 1989). A substantial relationship persists even when controlling for several of the potentially confounding factors in this association. However, relatively little evidence is available about the physiological or behavioral mechanisms linking short birth spacing and child health or about confounding socioeconomic factors. Considerably more research is needed before we can draw definitive conclusions about the reasons for or causal nature of this association or its magnitude.

EFFECTS OF UNWANTED PREGNANCY

The potential risks to a child's health of being born as the result of an unwanted pregnancy may be large. However, there is little direct evidence available on the subject, because distinguishing an unwanted from a wanted birth requires the measurement of attitudinal information about a couple's preferences and plans prior to conception. This information is sometimes not collected, and, when it is, it is usually measured after the birth, making its validity questionable. Tabulations from survey data, using retrospective reports of the wantedness status of births, do not show a consistent association between unwanted pregnancies and higher mortality risks.

However, there is limited evidence from other sources suggesting that children born as a result of unwanted pregnancies are likely to experience greater health and psychological problems. Scrimshaw (1978) reviews anthropological research and suggests that parents are less likely or less able to take adequate care of children born as a result of unwanted pregnancies. There is evidence of the possibility of selective parental neglect from South Asia, where there is a strong preference for male children. The results of several studies (Simmons et al.,

1982; Das Gupta, 1987; D'Souza and Chen, 1980; Bairagi, 1986; Chen et al., 1981) indicate that the higher mortality rates experienced by girls are due to poorer nutritional status and poorer care for girls who become ill. Weller et al. (1987) use survey data from the United States to show that women are not as likely to take adequate care of themselves during an unplanned pregnancy compared with a planned pregnancy. A study in Czechoslovakia by David et al. (1988) indicates that children whose mothers were denied requests for abortion suffer from a significantly higher incidence of psychological and developmental problems than other children. It is difficult to determine how applicable the findings of these last two studies are to families in contemporary developing countries. Nonetheless, this evidence suggests that children born as a result of unwanted pregnancies may be at higher risk. Grossman and Jacobowitz's results (1981) suggest that legalization of abortion in the United States may have contributed to the decline in infant mortality by reducing the incidence of unwanted pregnancies.

EFFECTS OF MATERNAL HEALTH CONDITIONS

Although the fetus is well protected from most infections, there are maternal infections, mostly viral, and other conditions that can affect the fetus. The effect of maternal viral infection on infant and child health is a serious concern with the spread of HIV, especially among populations in sub-Saharan Africa, where the disease affects many women and children. Other maternal behaviors also put infants at greater risk, specifically smoking, drug use, and alcohol abuse.

A recent report of the National Research Council (Turner et al., 1989) estimates the probability of HIV transmission from mother to infant is in the range of 30 to 50 percent. While considerable work on perinatal transmission of HIV remains to be done, the report also notes that some studies suggest that the risk of transmission is higher for infants born to mothers showing symptoms of HIV infection during pregnancy and those showing evidence of immunosuppression. HIV can also be transmitted from mother to infant via breast milk (Weinbreck et al., 1988).

Other important viral agents that may be passed from mother to fetus are toxoplasmosis, cytomegalovirus (CMV), rubella, hepatitis B virus, and herpes simplex. CMV and herpes simplex virus have been associated with fetal death, prematurity, intrauterine growth retardation, malformations, congenital infection, acute postnatal infection, and persistent postnatal infection. Rubella is associated with all of these except acute postnatal infection. Hepatitis B virus, which is endemic in Southeast Asia and other developing countries, has been linked to prematurity and fetal and neonatal infectious diseases (Overall, 1987).

Exposure to risks of sexually transmitted diseases and other genitourinary infections may be more likely among young women. Efiong and Banjoko (1975) found syphilis in 7 of 95 women in their first pregnancies younger than 16 in urban Nigeria, compared with none in 100 older women in their first pregnancies selected as controls. A prospective study in Sierra Leone found that pregnant women under age 20 were more likely to have both urinary and genital tract infections in pregnancy than were older pregnant women (World Health Organization, 1981).

Nonviral maternal infections are less likely to cross the placenta, but they may still affect the fetus before or during labor, especially if the membranes have ruptured prematurely. Infants born after premature rupture of the membranes are at increased risk of neonatal infections and respiratory distress syndrome.

Maternal parasite, fungal, and bacterial infections that can affect the fetus include malaria, syphilis, and tuberculosis. In general, congenital infections may produce symptoms at birth, but in the majority of cases they first produce symptoms after some months. Even a congenital infection that is not itself a direct cause of infant deaths may leave the infant more susceptible to later infection.

MINIMIZING THE RISKS OF CHILD DEATH

As discussed above, assessing the potential impact of changes in reproductive patterns for child survival is complicated because there is not yet sufficient evidence to determine how much of the observed association is actually causal. Furthermore, the potential impact of fertility changes is likely to differ significantly, depending on whether one is considering the impact on individual children, on individual families, or on the mortality experience of the population as a whole. Although it should be clear by now that more information is needed to determine exactly how (and how much) changes in reproduction may affect child health, in this section and the next we attempt to provide estimates of the possible size of the effects of reproductive change on individual children and families in developing countries, based on currently available information.

Risks to Individual Children

Our estimates are based on the Hobcraft (1987) analysis of 18 developing countries and reflect averages across these countries. These estimates are intended to illustrate the potential implications of the Hobcraft results and those of similar analyses. If one assumes that the relationships between child mortality and reproductive variables observed in the Hobcraft analysis are causal, our calculations indicate the actual reductions in mortality risks for children and families that could be brought about by changes in reproductive patterns. In fact, it is likely that these figures are overestimates of the true causal effect.

First, we use data from the 18 countries in Hobcraft's (1987) study to estimate an average child's probability of survival if he is born to a mother with a "better" reproductive history compared with an average child who was born to a mother with a "worse" reproductive history. It is important to keep in mind when considering these results that many less-than-optimal reproductive patterns (such as very close child spacing) are not common in many countries, as we discuss further in Chapter 6. The estimates described here apply to risks for individual children, not to population-level mortality rates, which are affected by the distribution of maternal age, birth order, and birth spacing in the population. The issue of effects on population-level mortality rates is discussed in Chapter 6 and 7.

In Table 5.2 we present estimated mortality rates from birth to age 2 for children born to women with "better" and "worse" spacing patterns, averaged across 18 developing countries separately for teenage and older mothers. We have defined the reproductive pattern that is better for a child as having no birth either in the two years before or in the two years after his own birth. The "poor" spacing pattern is defined as having one birth in the two years before the index child's birth and one birth in the two years afterward. Since all women who have children must, of course, have a first birth, we present these tabulations for children who are second or higher-order births. For purposes of comparison, we also assume that the previously born child for both categories of reproductive histories has survived to the index child's birth.

Children born to mothers ages 20 to 34 who have a better spacing pattern have a mortality rate of 67 deaths per 1,000 live births for 0- to 2-year-olds, which is almost half the rate for children born to women of the same age with a poor spacing pattern, and about 41 percent of the rate for children born to teenage mothers with a poor spacing pattern. It is clear from these figures, that, if the observed associations are causal, the potential gains to parents from improving spacing patterns and delaying childbearing until their twenties may be quite large, in terms of maximizing the survival chances for each of their children.

Risks to Families

Finally, we consider the risk to individual families of having a child die, given different mortality levels and different reproductive patterns. These results, shown in Table 5.3, are based on the same analysis (Hobcraft, 1987) discussed for Table 5.2 and are subject to the same caveats about causality and interpretation.

It is important to note that the figures in Table 5.3 are from a simulation based on several assumptions and reflect average risks across results from 18 developing countries. Thus, they do not reflect the experience of families in any country. Like the figures in Table 5.2, their purpose is illustrative. The estimates show, for a group of 100 families, how many of their children would die before they reached their fifth birthday. The average number is obviously affected by the prevailing child mortality rate, and we have therefore carried out the simulation for three arbitrary baseline levels of mortality: 50, 100, and 150 deaths per 1,000 live births. The baseline levels of mortality reflect the risk of dying between birth and age 5 for children with the lowest risk in the study population, i.e., children

TABLE 5.2 Estimated Average Mortality Rates for Second- and Higher-Order Children to Women With Different Reproductive Patterns

	Better Spacing Pattern	Poor Spacing Pattern
Teenage Mothers	92	165
Mothers Ages 20 to 34	67	120

Note: "Better" spacing pattern means that there were no births either in the 24 months before the index child or in the two years subsequent to the child's birth. "Poor" spacing pattern means that there was at least one birth during the 24 months before the index child and one birth in the two years after the index child's birth. For this comparison, in both cases, we assume the previous child survived.

Source: Hobcraft (1987:Table 13).

TABLE 5.3 Estimated Average Number of Child Deaths Experienced by Families Under Different Conditions, Per 100 Families

Number of Children Ever Born	Baseline Child Mortality Rate					
	50/1,000 Deaths		100/1,000 Deaths		150/1,000 Deaths	
	Closely Spaced	Well Spaced	Closely Spaced	Well Spaced	Closely Spaced	Well Spaced
4-child family	45	23	92	45	142	68
6-child family	70	33	144	65	222	98
9-child family	112	50	232	100	358	150

Source: Calculations based on figures in Hobcraft (1987:Table 1).

who are born at orders 2 or 3, who are well-spaced, and whose older siblings survived. We show simulations for families with 4, 6, and 9 children, because families who have more children are obviously going to be at greater risk of experiencing a child death, simply because they have more children. Estimates are shown separately for families in which all children are poorly spaced (birth intervals are all less than two years in length) and in which all children are well spaced (birth intervals are greater than two years in length).

The figures in Table 5.3 indicate that if the associations between reproductive variables and child survival are causal, families who space their children well are likely to loose fewer children than families who do not. For example, for a six-child family, the average number of child deaths experienced by families with well-spaced births is roughly half that for families with poorly spaced births.

APPENDIX TABLE 5.A Studies of Infant and Child Health

Study	Location and Type of Data	Dependent Variable	Type of Analysis, Controls
Aaby, Bukh, Lisse, and Smits, 1984	Guinea-Bissau; census and health data	Incidence and case fatality; rate of measles	Tabulations by HHC, A, CC, NS, E, SES
Bean, Mineau, and Anderton, 1987	United States; nineteenth-century Mormons, population-based longitudinal data	Infant mortality	Logit regression; controls: PBI, PCS, MA, MAM, PD, PSBI, BO, R
Bijur, Golding, and Kurzon, 1988	Great Britain; longitudinal data	Accident frequency	Logit regression; controls: HHC, SES, MMI, CHC
Boerma and van Vianen, 1984	Kenya; population-based longitudinal data	Mortality during first week, after the first week to 11 months, 12-23 months; birth-weight; mean weight and height at selected ages	Log-linear regression; controls: PBI, BO, MA. Lifetable by SBI and tabulations of BW and mean weight and height by PBI and SBI
Cantrelle and Leridon, 1971	Senegal; longitudinal data	Duration of breastfeeding; infant and child mortality; fertility	Tabulations by SSC, S, BO, M, MB, BF, PCS, PSBI, PBI
Chen, Hug, and D'Souza, 1981	Bangladesh; population-based longitudinal data	Mortality during the first month, 1-11 months, 1-4 years, 5-14 years, 15-44 years, 45-64 years, and 65+ years; nutritional status; morbidity; diarrhea treatment	Tabulations by A and S

APPENDIX TABLE 5.A Continued

Study	Location and Type of Data	Dependent Variable	Type of Analysis, Controls
Clark, 1981	Guatemala; population-based longitudinal data, cross-sectional socio-economic survey	Infant growth (change in weight between birth and six months, six and twelve months, birth and twelve months)	OLS regression; controls: SES, BF, SF, R, MW, MH, BO, MA, SB, PBI, HHC, S, BW
Cleland and Sathar, 1984	Pakistan; WFS—retrospective fertility history	Mortality during first month, 1-11 months, 12-23 months, 24-59 months.	Log-linear regression; controls: PBI, PCS, SES, R, S, BO, MA, PSBI, PI, BF, SBI
Costello, 1986	Uganda; Household survey, retrospective fertility history, medical data	Nutritional status	OLS Regression; controls: MA, MP, ML, PP, PL, P, L ME, MS, MAM, MG, R, SES
DaVanzo, Butz, and Habicht, 1983	Malaysia; Malaysian family life survey-retrospective fertility history	Mortality during first week, 8-28 days, 2-6 months, 7-11 months, 0-11 months	OLS and logit regression; controls: MA, PSBI, SB, PBI, S, BW, BO, BF, SES, YB, HHC, D, E, R
DaVanzo, Habicht, and Butz, 1984	Malaysia; Malaysian family life survey-retrospective fertility history	Birthweight	Logit, OLS, and variance-components least squares regression; controls: S, FB, MA, AM, PSBI, PBI, SES, DN, R, E, YB
Doyle, Morley Woodland, and Cole, 1978	Nigeria; population-based longitudinal data	Birth interval; birthweight; mean growth	Tabulations by BO, PCS, PCCS, SCS, PBI, SBI, K
D'Souza and Chen, 1980	Bangladesh; population-based longitudinal data	Infant and child mortality; mortality during 5-14, 15-44, 45-64 and 65+ years	Tabulations by YB, S, MB, CD
Fedrick, and Adelstein, 1973	Great Britain; cross-sectional perinatal mortality survey	Stillbirths; neonatal mortality; birthweight	Tabulations by PBI, SES, MA, CD, PCS

APPENDIX TABLE 5.A Continued

Study	Location and Type of Data	Dependent Variable	Type of Analysis, Controls
Fleming and Gray, 1988a	India; Narangwal Nutrition and Health Intervention Project, longitudinal data	Risk of mal-nutrition at selected ages.	Logit regression; controls: SBI, S, C, NS
Fleming and Gray, 1988b	India; Narangwal Nutrition and Health Inter-vention Project, longitudinal data	Birthweight; infant and child growth.	Logit regression; controls: S, C, PBI, BO, PCS
Fortney and Higgins, 1984	Iran; hospital-based data	Infant mortality before the mother's dis-charge from the hospital; birthweight	Logit regression; controls: PBI, BO, MA
Gubhaju, 1986	Nepal; WFS—retrospective fertility history	Infant and child mortality PCS, SES, R, YB	Logit regression; controls: BO, MA, S, PBI,
Hobcraft, 1987	34 countries; WFS—retrospective fertility histories	Mortality during first month, 1-11 months, 12-23 months, 24-59 months, 0-4 years	Log-linear regression; controls: PBI, SBI, BO, MA, S, SES; tabulations by family formation patterns (classification based on MA, BO, PBI, SBI)
Hobcraft, McDonald, and Rutstein, 1985a	39 countries; WFS—retrospective fertility histories	Mortality during first month, 1-11 months, 12-23 months 24-59 months	Log-linear regression; controls: PBI, SBI, BO, MA, S, SES
Knodel and Hermalin, 1984	Germany; nineteenth-century German villages, population-based longitudinal data	Mortality during first month, 1-11 months, 0-11 months, 12-59 months	Multiple classification analysis; tabulations by MA, BO, SS, PBI, PCS; controls: MA, PBI, R, PD

APPENDIX TABLE 5.A Continued

Study	Location and Type of Data	Dependent Variable	Type of Analysis, Controls
Koenig, Phillips, Campbell, and D'Souza, 1988	Bangladesh; population-based longitudinal data	Mortality during first month, 1-11 months, 12-23 months, 24-59 months	Hazard model; controls: S, MA, BO, SES, PBI, SBI
Palloni and Millman, 1986	12 Latin American countries; WFS—retrospective fertility histories	Mortality during 1-2 months, 3-5 months, 6-11 months, 12-59 months	Logit regression; controls: SES, MA, R, S, MB, SB, BO, BF, PBI, SBI
Pebley, Knodel, and Hermalin, 1988	Germany; nineteenth-century German villages, population-based longitudinal data	Infant mortality by birth rank SES, R, PD	Logit regression; controls: PCS, PBI, MA,
Pebley and Stupp, 1987	Guatemala; female life history survey, cross-sectional socio-economic survey	Infant and child mortality	Hazard model; controls: MA, BO, S, D, PCS, SES, YB, PBI, SBI, BF
Rosenzweig and Schultz, 1983	United States; national natality followback surveys, local area price, health, and labor force data	Birthweight	Two-stage least squares regression; controls: first stage— SES, R, HE, HDFP, PR, HFP, DP, J, E, UE, HB, ST; second stage—DD, SM, PAR, MA, E
Rutstein, 1983	41 countries; WFS—retrospective birth histories	Mortality during first month, 1-11 months, 0-11 months, 12-23 months, 24-59 months	Tabulations by YB, S, MA, BO, PBI, PCS, MB
Weller, Eberstein, and Bailey, 1987	United States; cross-sectional natality survey	Pregnancy wantedness measured by two indicators— cigarette smoking and timing of prenatal care	Logit regression; controls: E, SES, R, BO

APPENDIX TABLE 5.A Continued

Study	Location and Type of Data	Dependent Variable	Type of Analysis, Controls
Wolfers and Scrimshaw, 1975	Ecuador; retrospective fertility and sexual union histories	Birth interval length; pregnancy outcome; mortality during the first month, 1-11 months, 0-11 months, 12-23 months, 24-59 months	Tabulations by MA, BO, YB, PBI, SBI, PCS, PSBI

Note: Hobcraft et. al. (1985) presents regression estimates for 35 of the 39 countries included in the discussion. Hobcraft (1987) reviews findings for 34 of the 35 countries included in the regression analyses of Hobcraft et. al. (1985) and presents new analyses for 18 of the 34 countries by family formation patterns.

Key to Abbreviations

A	age group
AM	mother's age at menarche
BF	breastfeeding
BO	birth or pregnancy order
BW	birthweight
C	caste
CC	clustering of cases
CD	cause of death
CHC	child characteristics, such as aggression, overactivity, independence
D	type of delivery
DD	number of months pregnant before mother consulted a doctor or nurse
DN	distance to nurse
DP	number of doctors and OB-GYNs per capita
E	ethnicity
FB	first birth
HB	hospital beds per capita
HDFP	number of health departments with family planning services per capita
HE	local government health and hospital expenditures
HFP	number of hospitals with family planning services per capita
HHC	household composition
J	percentage of persons employed in manufacturing, service, or government jobs
K	history of kwashiorkor
L	currently breastfeeding
M	month of birth
MA	maternal age
MAM	mother's age at marriage
MB	multiple births
ME	menstruating
MG	presence of malaria or gonorrhea
MH	mother's height

ML	months breastfeeding
MMI	maternal malaise inventory, a measure of the psychological well-being of the mother
MP	months pregnant
MS	marital status
MW	mother's weight
NS	nutritional status
P	currently pregnant
PAR	number of live births born to mother
PBI	previous birth or pregnancy interval
PCCS	survival of a child prior to the preceding child
PCS	survival of previous child
PI	prior interval (birth interval immediately prior to the preceding interval)
PD	previous infant deaths
PL	months breastfeeding/months exposed to conception
PP	months pregnant/months exposed to conception
PR	cigarette and milk prices
PSBI	proportion of other pregnancy intervals that are short or average of birth intervals
R	urban/rural residence or region
S	sex of child
SB	proportion or number of stillbirths
SBI	subsequent birth interval
SCS	survival of subsequent child
SES	education, income, occupation, housing characteristics
SF	supplementary food
SM	number of cigarettes smoked per day by mother while pregnant
SS	sibship size
SSC	survival status of the index child
ST	sales tax on cigarettes
UE	general and female unemployment rate
YB	year of birth

6

Changes in Reproductive Patterns

Previous chapters of this report focused on the consequences of different aspects of reproductive patterns for the health of women and children as individuals. We examined the relationships between maternal age, birth spacing, and birth order and the health of individual women and children. The health of women, we concluded, can be improved by reducing the number of births and especially by reducing high-risk births, specifically those of high-parity and to very young and older women. The health of individual children can also be improved by reducing high-risk births, specifically births to very young women and births occurring less than 24 months after a previous birth. In this chapter we change the focus of our attention and examine the degree to which reproductive patterns vary among developing countries and the extent to which these patterns have changed as societies move through demographic transition.

This chapter reviews evidence of changes in the proportions of high-risk births occurring in countries as their levels of fertility decline. As fertility in a society declines, other aspects of the society's pattern of reproduction may also change. For example, women may be more likely to compress their childbearing by delaying their first birth, having births closer together, and having their last birth at a younger age. This was what happened in South Korea (Donaldson and Nichols, 1978). Such changes in the timing, spacing, and numbers of births in a society change the proportion of high-risk births and thus affect the health of the women and children in that society.

Our review of reproductive patterns in the developing world begins with an examination of changes in birth order distributions that have occurred in countries in which fertility has declined. We then examine evidence of changes in ages when mothers begin and when they complete childbearing as fertility declines in a society. We then examine patterns and trends in birth spacing and the relationship between contraceptive use and abortion. Finally, we examine how changes in reproductive patterns affect mortality rates.

Most of the evidence presented in this chapter comes from three large-scale survey research projects supported by the Agency for International Development: the World Fertility Survey (WFS), the Contraceptive Prevalence Surveys (CPS), and the Demographic and Health Surveys (DHS). Additional information comes from other cross-sectional surveys and from national vital registration systems. Unfortunately, comparable data from the same set of countries are not always available, and the countries for which data are available are not necessarily representative of the experiences of the developing world. However, the available data show considerable variation among societies in reproductive patterns and allow us to illustrate the experience of many developing countries as their reproductive patterns change. The increasing availability of more than one national sample survey of fertility in many developing countries will make it easier for future studies to examine changes in reproductive patterns. At the same time, it should be recognized that one of the factors that can contribute to a fertility decline and changing reproductive patterns is the level of infant mortality, so that there are reciprocal effects.

The rates for a given event in a population depend on the rates for that event in each subgroup and the relative size of that subgroup in the population. For example, the overall infant mortality rate may be thought of as resulting from the infant mortality rates applying to each birth order and the proportion of births by birth order. The emphasis in this chapter, however, is on the distribution of births by birth order, mother's age, and birth interval, and how these are likely to change as fertility declines.

In order to gauge how the infant mortality rate will change with changing reproductive patterns, it is necessary to know the level of infant mortality associated with each subgroup. At the same time, it should be recognized that these subgroup rates may themselves change as reproductive patterns vary. The variations in infant mortality rates associated with different levels of subgroup characteristics provide some indication of the changes that might result from changing reproductive patterns. At the same time, it should be noted that the exact amount of change will also depend on the trends in the group-specific infant mortality rates.

The emphasis in this chapter is on the distributions of births in populations, and not on the probability of births to individuals or subgroups or how these distributions are likely to change as fertility declines. For example, a decline in births to older women may mean that an increased proportion of all births will occur to younger women, even if birth rates decline for both young and older women. It is virtually certain, for example, that lower fertility will result in a decrease in the proportion of higher-order births and a corresponding increase in the proportion of first births. Lower fertility probably will lead to a decrease in the proportion of births to older women, but it is not clear what effect lower fertility will have on the proportion of births to very young women. There are limited grounds on which a prediction can be made about possible changes in the distribution of birth intervals. Several scenarios are possible. For example, if there is a reduction in breastfeeding without a corresponding increase in contraceptive use as fertility declines, birth intervals will become shorter. Average interval length could also decrease as a result of changes in the birth order distribution. Intervals between higher-order births are often longer than between lower-order births, so fertility declines that reduce higher-order births and concentrate births among lower orders could result in shorter average interval lengths. However, if contraceptive use for spacing births increases without a corresponding decrease in breastfeeding, the length of intervals may increase as fertility declines. These changes may occur simultaneously, adding to the difficulty of predicting the effect of changing fertility on the length of birth intervals. However, since potential changes in the distributions of high-risk births may significantly affect the health of women and children in a society, these changes need to be understood.

FERTILITY DECLINES AND BIRTH ORDER DISTRIBUTION

Total fertility rates in the developing world have declined from an estimated average of 6.1 during the first half of the 1950s to an estimated average of 4.1 during the first half of the 1980s (United Nations, 1988c). Significant declines in total fertility rates have occurred throughout Latin America and Asia, as is well known. However, declines in total fertility rates have not taken place throughout the entire developing world: for example, although the fertility decline in China has been extraordinary, the total fertility rates in sub-Saharan African countries are estimated by the United Nations (1988c) to have increased slightly.

As the total fertility rate of a population declines, the proportion of all births that are first births increases and the proportion of higher-order births (fifth and higher births) decreases. This is illustrated in Table 6.1, which shows changes in the distribution of first and higher-order births for 11 countries that have experienced significant fertility declines and that the United Nations judges to have reasonably complete vital registration data.

In each case, the proportion of all births that are of order 1 increased substantially, more than doubling in some countries, and the proportion of higher-order births decreased. For example, in Malaysia the proportion of first births increased from 12 to 26 percent, and the proportion of fifth- and higher-order births decreased from 41 to 22 percent. These changes decrease the number of high-risk, higher-order births and increase the proportion of high-risk first births. We will return to the effects such distributional changes have on measures of health and mortality at the end of the chapter.

TABLE 6.1 Change in the Order Distribution of Births in Selected Countries Over the Course of Fertility Declines by Percentage Decline in Total Fertility Rates.

Country	Proportion of All Births of Order 1		Proportion of all Births of Order 5+		Percent decline in TFR
	1960s	1970s-1980	1960s	1970s-1980	
Singapore	.23	.44	.33	.02	65
Hong Kong	.25	.43	.23	.04	64
Barbados	.22	.40	.35	.10	54
Mauritius	.18	.36	.36	.11	52
Costa Rica	.18	.32	.45	.17	50
Chile	.25	.41	.31	.09	49
Trinidad and Tobago	.19	.32	.37	.19	43
Puerto Rico	.27	.32	.27	.10	42
Panama	.21	.29	.35	.22	42
Malaysia	.12	.26	.41	.22	42
Fiji	.23	.35	.36	.13	41

Source: *United Nations Demographic Yearbook*, various years.

MATERNAL AGES AT CHILDBEARING

Because very young and older maternal ages are associated with increased risk for both women and children, we are interested in the changes that are likely to take place as fertility declines in the ages at which women begin and end childbearing. There is considerable information on the age at which women begin childbearing. Information on age at completion of childbearing is more limited, because measuring this requires that cohorts have completed childbearing. However, we can show changes in the proportion of births to women over age 35 in some developing countries that have experienced declines in fertility.

Age at first birth has been rising in many developing countries. Trussell and Reinis (1989) have estimated mean ages at first birth by age groups for the 40 developing countries participating in the WFS. It is difficult to be certain that these data reflect change over time because of the tendency for women, especially older women, not to report their first birth if it did not survive. The Trussell and Reinis estimates, which are presented in Table 6.2, show increases in age at first birth in most of the countries that have experienced declines in total fertility. By comparing the average at first birth of the youngest with that of the oldest groups, we can estimate the extent to which change has taken place. For example, in

TABLE 6.2 Mean Age at First Birth, by Age

Country	Age at Time of Survey					
	20-24	25-29	30-34	35-39	40-44	45-49
Africa						
Benin	21.0	20.5	20.4	20.4	21.1	21.6
Cameroon	19.6	20.1	19.9	20.6	20.7	22.0
Egypt	21.7	22.2	20.5	20.0	20.0	19.9
Ghana	20.4	20.7	20.6	20.5	21.2	21.2
Ivory Coast	19.0	19.4	19.2	19.9	20.1	20.4
Kenya	19.9	19.6	19.2	19.7	20.0	21.3
Lesotho	20.9	21.2	21.4	21.6	21.9	21.5
Mauritania	20.9	19.6	18.8	20.0	20.7	21.1
Morocco	22.5	21.4	20.4	19.5	19.9	19.5
Nigeria	20.0	20.2	20.2	20.9	22.5	22.9
Senegal	19.4	19.4	18.3	18.5	18.7	19.4
Sudan (North)	20.7	20.1	19.4	20.7	20.4	21.8
Tunisia	24.8	24.2	22.3	22.0	22.1	22.7
Asia and the Pacific						
Bangladesh	17.5	17.1	17.1	17.4	17.9	18.1
Fiji	23.2	22.4	20.9	20.6	20.4	20.7
Indonesia	21.0	20.5	19.8	19.6	20.1	20.7
Jordan	20.2	20.5	20.1	20.2	20.1	19.7
Korea	25.1	24.1	24.2	22.7	21.8	20.7
Malaysia	24.1	23.5	22.0	20.9	20.8	20.4
Nepal	21.0	20.8	20.8	21.5	21.7	22.0
Pakistan	20.1	20.6	19.9	19.8	19.1	19.4
Philippines	23.4	23.1	23.1	22.5	22.4	23.0
Sri Lanka	25.8	25.6	22.9	22.8	21.6	21.6
Syria	22.6	21.8	21.1	22.0	22.0	22.0
Thailand	22.9	23.0	22.2	22.7	22.4	22.4
Turkey	21.8	20.9	20.6	19.9	20.4	20.8
Yemen Arabic Republic	19.9	19.9	20.9	21.4	22.3	24.1
Caribbean and Latin America						
Colombia	22.6	22.4	21.6	21.7	22.0	22.5
Costa Rica	22.4	22.9	21.9	21.7	21.9	22.8
Dominican Republic	21.2	20.3	20.7	20.2	20.3	21.3
Ecuador	22.7	22.4	21.5	21.3	21.3	22.4
Guyana	21.6	21.1	20.4	20.4	20.1	20.7
Haiti	24.9	23.8	23.5	23.4	22.0	24.1
Jamaica	19.5	20.5	19.8	20.3	21.5	21.7
Mexico	21.8	21.8	21.3	21.2	21.1	21.5
Panama	22.7	22.1	21.2	21.2	21.1	21.2
Paraguay	23.1	22.5	22.3	22.4	21.4	22.0
Peru	22.8	22.1	22.0	21.4	21.5	21.9
Trinidad and Tobago	22.6	23.1	22.3	21.6	20.7	20.8
Venezuela	22.4	22.2	21.8	21.3	21.4	n.a.

Source: Trussell and Reinis (1989). Mean ages are based on data derived from the World Fertility Surveys and are estimated based on statistical models developed by Coale and McNeil (1972) and Rodriguez and Trussell (1980).

Malaysia women ages 45-49 were on average 20.4 when they had their first birth. Trussell and Reinis's estimates show that, in Africa, only Egypt, Morocco, and Tunisia experienced a rise in the mean age at first birth. In Asia and the Pacific, one sees more increases in the estimated mean age at first birth, especially in countries with significant fertility declines, such as Korea and Malaysia. In the Caribbean and Latin America, however, the mean age at first birth has changed relatively little, even though many of the countries in this region have experienced notable declines in fertility.

Data on changes in age at last birth are more difficult to obtain because cohorts of women must have completed their fertility in order for age at the last birth to be measured accurately. McDonald (1984) estimated the mean age at last birth for 30 countries for women who were ages 40-49 at the time the data were collected. Mean ages at last birth for these women ranged from 31.5 for Indians in Guyana to 38.4 in Kenya. Unfortunately, there are no later cohorts for comparison.

Another way to see if changes have occurred in the age pattern of childbearing is to examine the proportion of all births occurring to young and older women at two different times. Table 6.3 shows proportions of births to younger women (under 20) and older women (over 35) at two time periods in 11 developing countries that have experienced significant declines in fertility. The proportion of births to women ages 35 and older declined in all these countries. Declines were substantial in some cases—from 20 to 6 percent in Hong Kong—and marginal in

TABLE 6.3 Changes in the Distribution of Births by Maternal Age in Selected Countries Over the Course of Fertility Decline by Percent Decline in Total Fertility Rates Between 1960 and 1980

Country	Proportion of All Births to Women Under 20		Proportion of All Births to Women 35+		Percent Decline in TFR
	1960s	1970s-1980	1960s	1970s-1980	
Singapore	.08	.04	.14	.05	65
Hong Kong	.05	.04	.20	.06	64
Barbados	.21	.25	.15	.06	54
Mauritius	.13	.14	.15	.07	52
Costa Rica	.13	.20	.18	.09	50
Chile	.12	.17	.17	.09	49
Trinidad and Tobago	.17	.19	.11	.08	43
Puerto Rico	.18	.18	.11	.07	42
Panama	.18	.20	.11	.09	42
Malaysia	.11	.07	.14	.13	42
Fiji	.13	.11	.12	.08	41

Source: *United Nations Demographic Yearbook*, various years.

others, especially in those countries with a relatively low proportion of births to older women in the earlier time period, such as Panama. Those countries with the greatest fertility declines all experienced a substantial drop in the proportions of births to women ages 35 and older. The proportion of births to women younger than age 20 increased in 6 of the 11 populations as their fertility declined.

Delaying age at first birth can benefit the health of women and their children, particularly for women who might begin childbearing at very young ages. The data on ages at which women begin childbearing reviewed above indicate that, in a number of countries, fertility declines have also been accompanied by increasing ages at first birth. A decrease in the proportion of births to older women is also related to declines in fertility. This change in reproductive pattern has probably benefited the health of women and children in these populations.

SPACING OF BIRTHS

As shown in Chapter 5, births following a previous birth by less than 24 months are associated with increased risk in many developing countries, in developed countries, and in high-mortality historical populations. Although scientists have not yet specified the precise mechanisms involved in these relationships, the association is so widespread that it is prudent to be concerned about the potential effects on infant health of short birth intervals.

There is limited evidence regarding the relationship between changes in the proportion of short birth intervals (less than two years) in a population and changes in levels of fertility. Table 6.4 presents Hobcraft's (1987) estimates for 18 countries of the proportion of second- and higher-order births that followed the previous birth by less than 2 years during the 10 years preceding the WFS survey. This table presents a cross-sectional view of countries at different stages in the demographic transition. Kenya and Jordan, the countries with the highest total fertility rates, have a high proportion of short birth intervals. However, among the other countries, those with lower levels of fertility tend to have higher proportions of short birth intervals than those with higher levels of fertility. Over half the births in Costa Rica occurred less than two years after the previous birth, and their total fertility rate of 3.8 is relatively low. In comparison, 37 percent of births in Bangladesh followed within two years of a previous birth, while the total fertility rate was 6.1.

If an increase in short intervals occurs when fertility declines, then there are reasons to be concerned about the increased risk to infants associated with increases in the proportion of short birth intervals. However, this cross-sectional perspective may be an incomplete or inaccurate view of the relationship between changes in birth spacing and fertility declines.

Published data on changes in the proportion of short birth intervals in populations experiencing declines in fertility are surprisingly limited. Table 6.5 presents data from 10 countries in which both birth interval data and total fertility rates are

TABLE 6.4 Proportion of Births of Orders Two and Above That Occurred Less Than Two Years After the Previous Birth and Total Fertility Rates for the Five-Year Period Prior to the Survey

Country (Survey year)	Proportion with preceding Interval < 2 Years	Total Fertility Rate
Kenya (1977-1978)	.40	8.2
Jordan (1976)	.54	7.8
Senegal (1978)	.21	7.1
Cameroon (1978)	.32	6.3
Ivory Coast (1980-1981)	.29	6.3
Bangladesh (1975-1976)	.37	6.1
Morocco (1980)	.42	5.9
Lesotho (1977)	.20	5.6
Peru (1977-1978)	.44	5.5
Jamaica (1975-1976)	.48	5.0
Colombia (1976)	.53	4.6
Malaysia (1974)	.41	4.6
Thailand (1975)	.37	4.5
Panama (1975-1976)	.47	4.4
Korea (1974)	.22	4.2
Costa Rica (1976)	.53	3.8
Sri Lanka (1975)	.35	3.7
Trinidad and Tobago (1977)	.49	3.2

Sources: For intervals, Hobcraft (1987); for fertility rates, Goldman, Rutstein, and Singh (1985).

available for some point in the 1970s and some point in the 1980s. For two of these countries, Thailand and Taiwan, we also have data from the 1960s. In 8 of these 10 populations, the proportion of birth intervals of less than two years decreased as fertility levels dropped. These data are admittedly limited, but they do present a picture opposite from that given by cross-sectional data showing that the proportion of intervals that are short is negatively associated with total fertility rates over time. If birth intervals do lengthen as fertility levels decline, improvements in maternal and child health should occur. However, the increase in the proportion of short intervals in Senegal should be of concern to health officials and policy makers, particularly if this reflects emerging patterns in Africa. As data collected at more than one time become available for a larger number of countries, the relationship should become clearer.

Breastfeeding and postpartum abstinence are the primary traditional factors contributing to long interbirth intervals. Intensive unsupplemented breastfeeding postpones the return of ovulation (McNeilly, 1977), thus extending the length of birth intervals. Postpartum abstinence, which can have mean durations greater

TABLE 6.5 Changes in the Distribution of Births by Length of Preceding Interval and Total Fertility Rates (TFR) in Selected Countries

Country	1960s Proportion of intervals less than 24 months	TFR	1970s Proportion of intervals less than 24 months	TFR	1980s Proportion of intervals less than 24 months	TFR
Senegal			21	7.1	34	6.6^g
Ecuador			46	5.3	28	4.3^g
Peru			41	5.5	26	4.1^d
Mexico			49	6.1	28	3.8^e
Dominican Republic			54	5.7	25	3.7^d
Colombia			53	4.6	21	3.3^g
Trinidad and Tobago			49	3.2	17	3.1^g
Sri Lanka			35	3.7	19	2.7^g
Taiwan	37^a	5.1^b	49^a	3.4^c	53^a	2.6^f
Thailand	30^a	6.1	25^a	5.1^a	19^a	2.4^g

^{a} Closed intervals occurring within 12 months of survey. All other birth intervals are for the 10 years prior to the surveys.
^{b} 1963-1965.
^{c} 1971-1973.
^{d} 3 years prior to survey.
^{e} Year prior to survey.
^{f} 1978-1980.
^{g} 5 years preceding survey.

Sources: Senegal, Ecuador, Peru, Mexico, Dominican Republic, Colombia, Trinidad and Tobago, Sri Lanka: 1980s data provided by the Demographic and Health Survey project; 1970s data from the World Fertility Survey (A. Pebley). Taiwan: Data provided by A. Hermalin. Thailand: John Knodel and Kua Wongboonsin, "Birth Interval and Birth Order Distributions over Thailand's Fertility Transition." August, 1988. 1980 TFRs from *DHS Newsletter* except Taiwan.

than a year in some populations, is also an important influence on birth interval lengths in some countries. Table 6.6 presents estimates of mean durations of breastfeeding and postpartum abstinence by Singh and Ferry (1984) for 20 WFS countries. Mean durations of full (unsupplemented) breastfeeding range from 2.2 months in Kenya to 7.9 months in Mauritania. Mean duration of total breastfeeding is as high as 26.5 months in Bangladesh. Countries with longer intervals between births tend to be the countries in which durations of breastfeeding are longer. There is a wide range in periods of postpartum abstinence, with mean durations of more than a year in several countries.

In most developing countries, more women have breastfed than have used modern contraception; therefore declines in breastfeeding could greatly increase the proportion of short birth intervals (DaVanzo and Starbird, 1989). Accordingly, some experts have been concerned that breastfeeding in the developing

TABLE 6.6 Breastfeeding and Postpartum Abstinence in 20 Countries

Country	Mean Duration (months)			% of Mothers Who Ever Breastfeed
	Breastfeeding	Unsupplemented Breastfeeding	Postpartum Abstinence	
Bangladesh	26.5	n.a.	3.0	98
Benin	19.2	2.6	15.5	97
Lesotho	19.1	2.5	15.0	95
Ghana	17.9	4.5	10.0	92
Senegal	17.7	4.9	n.a.	98
Cameroon	17.5	5.1	13.9	98
Ivory Coast	17.5	5.0	13.1	98
Kenya	16.9	2.2	2.9	98
Egypt	16.3	7.4	n.a.	95
Sudan (North)	15.8	5.6	2.6	98
Mauritania	15.6	7.9	n.a.	98
Haiti	15.3	n.a.	6.5	96
Morocco	14.2	5.5	n.a.	94
Tunisia	14.0	6.2	1.6	95
Philippines	12.6	3.3	2.8	86
Syria	11.2	5.5	1.2	95
Paraguay	10.9	2.9	1.5	93
Yemen A.R.	10.6	4.5	2.8	92
Fiji	9.4	n.a.	5.1	87
Costa Rica	5.0	n.a.	1.3	75

Source: Singh and Ferry (1984:Table 5).

world has declined. Millman (1986), however, found variability in trends in breastfeeding practices among the populations she examined, with decreases in some populations, increases in some, and stability in patterns in others. She concludes that there is no evidence of systematic declines in levels of breastfeeding, although substantial declines have occurred in some countries, for example, Taiwan. However, data concerning breastfeeding trends are limited, and it is difficult to be certain that rapid changes in breastfeeding practice are not occurring.

Survey data from many countries indicate that many women desire to space their births. In Africa, spacing children has been a dominant reason for using contraception, although prevalence of modern contraception remains extremely low (London et al., 1985). In 17 Latin American and Caribbean countries for which WFS data are available, an average of 38 percent of women contracepting were doing so to delay their next birth, compared with 48 percent who were using contraception to prevent further childbearing (Cleland and Rutstein, 1986). Cross-national analyses of contraceptive use for spacing are difficult because no standard set of women has been asked questions about contraception for spacing, and the form of the questions concerning contraception for spacing has varied.

While a significant proportion of women apparently wish to space their births, there is a negative association between the two primary mechanisms affecting spacing, breastfeeding, and contraceptive use. Women who breastfeed are less likely than others to use contraception, and women who practice contraception are less likely to breastfeed (Millman, 1985; DaVanzo and Starbird, 1989). Pebley et al. (1985) found that the proportion of breastfeeding women using oral contraceptives was generally low, but not inconsequential. Gomez de Leon and Potter (1989) present evidence suggesting that many women may either perceive breastfeeding and contraceptive use to be incompatible or they substitute one for the other.

Births within 24 months of a previous birth are at increasing risk, but no clear picture emerges on the association between declining fertility and changes in the proportion of short birth intervals. The proportion of short intervals decreased as fertility declined in the six Latin American countries in Table 6.5, as was also the case in Sri Lanka and Thailand. However, the proportion of short intervals increased in Senegal and Taiwan. Trends in breastfeeding and contraceptive use for spacing are also not clear, but there is an inverse association between the two behaviors that influence spacing.

CONTRACEPTIVE USE AND INDUCED ABORTION

Abortion may be used when women wish to control fertility but do not practice contraception or when they experience a contraceptive failure. However, because of lack of data, it is impossible to estimate the incidence of abortion or the relationship between changes in contraceptive use and abortion in developing countries.

Three patterns of abortion and contraceptive use can be identified from the limited data available for countries moving from high to lower levels of fertility (Rogers, 1988). Abortion rates may increase during the early stages of the fertility transition, as women began to control their fertility and contraceptive use increases. This has been the experience in China, Singapore, and Taiwan, although a different pattern may take place in different cultural contexts. The second pattern was found in many countries of Western Europe and Japan, as the progression from high to low fertility combined with the assimilation of effective contraception was accompanied by a decline in abortion. A third pattern is characteristic of low-fertility countries in which the use of effective contraception is widespread, abortion is legal and available, and its use appears to be low. This is the current situation in England and Wales and the Netherlands. Overall then, the evidence suggests that the increased use of effective contraception can reduce the incidence of induced abortion, unless it is already low.

EFFECTS OF CHANGES IN REPRODUCTIVE PATTERNS ON MORTALITY RATES

It is clear that, as fertility declines, reproductive patterns may change in several ways simultaneously. The effect of changes in reproductive patterns on infant, child, and maternal mortality rates will depend on how pregnancies and births are distributed during the fertility decline among higher- and lower-risk groups (Bongaarts, 1987). For example, a decrease in the proportion of births occurring at high parities may reduce mortality rates, if everything else remains the same. An increase in the proportion of births that are first births, however, may increase mortality rates, holding everything else constant, because mortality risks associated with first births appear to be higher for both women and children than risks associated with second, third and fourth births. Data presented in this chapter suggest that, as the proportion of higher-order births declines during a fertility transition, the proportion of first births may increase. Since both higher-order births and first births have greater mortality risks, the net effect of a change in the distribution of births by birth order during a fertility decline will depend on the relative size of the mortality risk for firstborns and for higher-order births, as well as the extent of the redistribution of births among these parities.

This is another illustration of the fact that the overall infant mortality rate is the weighted average of the infant mortality rates operating for each subgroup. Several things follow from this: it is possible for the specific mortality rates for each birth order to decline over time, but for the overall rate to increase because of a higher proportion of first births at the second date. In addition, changes in the infant mortality rate are not necessarily associated with changes in the number of infant deaths. If there are fewer births over time, there will be fewer deaths, even if the infant mortality rate remains at the same level. This has implications for the demands made on the health infrastructure in providing care to women and children.

Using figures from Hobcraft (1987), Bongaarts (1987) has shown that because of shifts in the birth order distribution, a fertility decline may have very little effect on infant mortality rates, even when reducing the number of high-parity births that families have reduces the number of infant deaths they experience. This possibility is discussed in greater detail by Bongaarts (1988), Trussell (1988), and Potter (1988). As we note in Chapter 5, however, Hobcraft's (1987) results and those of other studies suggest that there is substantial variation among populations in the relative risks of mortality of first and higher-order births.

In a few countries, it appears that risks of infant and child mortality for first births are not substantially higher than those for second, third, and fourth births. If mortality risks rise with birth order in these populations, reducing the proportion of births at higher birth orders could therefore bring about significant reductions in infant mortality rates. The central point is that the likely effect of a fertility decline on mortality rates will depend on a country's particular situation and on the way its reproductive patterns change during the fertility transition.

A related issue concerns the potential for change in mortality rates caused by a change in fertility. The amount of change in mortality rates will depend on how common potentially detrimental reproductive patterns are in a population. For example, birth spacing patterns and the frequency of pregnancy at very young ages vary considerably in developing countries. The proportion of intervals that are very short is small in most countries in sub-Saharan Africa and South Asia. In these regions there is not much room to reduce this proportion further, as there is, for example, in Latin America. Rather, as fertility declines, the concern of policy makers should be to prevent an increase in the proportion of birth intervals that are detrimentally short by respecting traditional practices and by promoting breastfeeding and contraceptive use for spacing. Childbearing at very young ages is more common in some South Asian countries than elsewhere in the world, and therefore the scope for improving women's and children's health through delays in the age at first birth is greater in these countries.

CONCLUSION

As levels of fertility decline in developing countries, their patterns of reproduction also change. In particular, women may begin bearing children at later ages and complete childbearing at earlier ages, and the spacing between births may change. These changes in timing and spacing are likely to directly affect the health of women and children in these countries in addition to the direct benefits of having fewer children.

In many developing countries in which fertility has declined, age at marriage and age at first birth have increased. Delaying age at first birth is likely to benefit women and children, especially in societies in which childbearing begins at very young ages. Although published evidence on changes in birth spacing is surprisingly scarce, cross-sectional relationships between the proportion of short birth intervals and the total fertility rates of countries indicate that spacing tends to be closer in societies with lower fertility. However, in 8 of the 10 countries in which data on spacing are available for two or more times, the proportion of short intervals declined as fertility declined. While the available data indicate that changes in birth spacing are likely to occur as fertility declines, the direction of change remains unclear. Analysis of spacing using data from the Demographic and Health Surveys currently under way will give further indication of relationships between birth spacing and fertility declines.

Declining fertility does lead to changes in the distribution of births by birth order; most notably, the proportion of births that are first births, which are typically higher-risk births, increases. Because of the change in the birth order distribution and the different level of risk associated with different birth orders, the paradoxical situation can arise whereby aggregate measures of mortality, such as the infant mortality rate, can increase, although the mortality rate for each birth order may decrease. In addition, as fertility declines, the number of infant deaths will decline, even if the infant mortality rate does not change.

The overall health of a population may improve as fertility declines, both because of the direct and indirect effects discussed in this report, and because of factors such as improved nutrition and improved delivery of health care. Thus, the level of risk associated with first births or close birth spacing may decrease over time. As health and demographic data continue to be collected and compared with information from earlier surveys, the complex associations among the numerous factors influencing the health of women and children should be better understood.

7

Conclusions

Since World War II, there have been major improvements in the health of women and children in most developing countries. These improvements, however, have been unevenly distributed: they have been dramatic in some countries, moderate in others, and small in many countries, particularly the poorest countries of Africa and South Asia. Overall, the incidence of poor health and of infant, child, and maternal mortality remains unacceptably high throughout the developing world. Many developing countries have also experienced significant declines in fertility over the last 40 years. Other countries with the highest rates of infant, child, and maternal mortality also have high fertility rates. This report has examined the relationship between fertility and health during the course of this transition in fertility and mortality and has assessed the impact of changes in reproductive patterns on the health of women and children.

As discussed throughout the report, assessing the health effects of reproductive patterns and changes in them is not a straightforward task. First, as outlined in Chapter 2, the relationships between fertility and health are very complex. For this evaluation, we have focused on what we term *direct effects*, a subset of the possible associations between reproductive patterns and women's and children's health. For example, we hypothesize that child spacing directly affects child mortality through mechanisms such as maternal depletion. By contrast, an indirect effect could occur if mothers who space their children more closely were less likely to be able to work for pay and thus improve the economic status of their family. Other indirect relationships between fertility and health may be as important as the direct effects.

90

Second, the data on which studies cited in this report are based are often seriously deficient. For example, data on maternal health and mortality are scarce, and research examining the relationship between birth spacing and maternal mortality in developing countries has yet to be carried out. Most studies of contraceptive risks and benefits are based on data from industrialized countries, and conclusions about the safety of contraceptive use in developing countries must in part be made by extrapolation. Information on gestational age, birthweight, and maternal and infant nutritional status, which is necessary to sort out the association between birth spacing and child health, has been difficult to collect in developing countries. Furthermore, most data on which analyses of maternal and child health are based come from observational rather than experimental studies, a situation that complicates analytic designs, making it more difficult to draw inferences about causality.

Third, the limitations of the analytic strategies of many studies make firm conclusions difficult to draw. Many studies have not adequately considered alternative factors that may account for the observed relationships. Problems such as relevant, unmeasured influences and the joint operation of causal factors affect many studies of human behavior, but may be particularly troublesome in the associations discussed in this report because fertility and health are complex, interrelated processes. Few of the studies on which this report is based have attempted to deal with these issues in a comprehensive manner.

While the shortcomings of the evidence are clear and should be kept in mind, we believe that the available evidence is sufficient to draw important conclusions about how reproductive patterns affect women's and children's health.

REPRODUCTIVE PATTERNS AND WOMEN'S HEALTH: RISKS FOR INDIVIDUAL WOMEN

Maternal mortality has declined significantly in this century in the developed world. Some developing countries have also witnessed declines in maternal mortality because of improvements in prenatal care, better midwifery, widespread use of aseptic delivery procedures, the introduction of antibiotics, improvements in the provision of health services, and overall advances in women's social position and standard of living. These experiences provide unequivocal evidence that mortality and morbidity due to reproductive causes can be reduced. What role can changes in reproductive patterns play in this process?

It is clear that reductions in the number of pregnancies women have in their lifetimes and in the incidence of high-risk pregnancies will substantially reduce the risk of maternal mortality and morbidity for individual women. Furthermore, the positive effects of lower fertility and reductions in the frequency of high-risk pregnancies on women's health are likely to be greatest in populations in which fertility rates are high, health facilities are poor or unavailable, and the incidence of reproductive morbidity is high.

Each time they become pregnant, women face a risk of morbidity and mortality, and these risks are higher in societies in which health conditions are poor. A reduction in the number of times a woman becomes pregnant during her life will reduce her lifetime risk of dying from reproductive causes. If, in addition to reducing the total number of pregnancies she has, a woman uses contraception to avoid high-risk pregnancies, the beneficial effect will be reinforced. Pregnancies that are particularly high risks for women include those that occur when a woman has a previous gynecological or obstetrical illness or problem, such as postpartum hemorrhage, or has a preexisting health problem, such as diabetes, while she is pregnant.

In addition, pregnancies to very young and older women, and first- and higher-order pregnancies (fifth and higher-order) appear to be riskier than others. While first births cannot, of course, be avoided if a woman chooses to have children, the risks appear to be attenuated if the first birth is delayed beyond the high-risk early teenage years.

Risks Associated With Induced Abortion

Unsafe induced abortion is an important cause of reproductive morbidity and mortality. As noted in Chapter 3, unsafe induced abortion is a primary cause of maternal mortality. Family planning services have the potential to reduce abortion-related health problems by reducing unwanted pregnancies. Countries in which safe abortion is not available have the greatest obligation to provide all needed contraceptive and medical services to reduce unintended pregnancy and to treat the complications of unsafe abortion.

Contraceptive Risks and Benefits

According to a United Nations (1989) estimate, over 400 million women in developing countries are using some form of contraception. This diffusion of modern contraceptives has facilitated widespread regulation of fertility. The most important conclusion to be drawn from the extensive literature examining the noncontraceptive health risks and benefits of contraception is that risks associated with contraceptive use are significantly less than the risks associated with pregnancy and childbirth. This conclusion is especially true in many countries in the developing world where childbirth and pregnancy risks are high.

Although contraception in general is safer than pregnancy, it is nonetheless important to consider contraceptive risks and benefits in relation to the characteristics of different women. For example, to recall Chapter 4, decisions to use oral contraceptives should consider factors such as age and whether a woman smokes cigarettes, and decisions to use an intrauterine device should consider a woman's pattern of sexual activity. Both contraceptive needs and the risk-benefit profiles of women change over the course of their reproductive lives. Information about risks and benefits, including information on contraceptive efficacy, at different life-cycle stages is necessary for informed decision making and for safer, more effective contraceptive practice.

An ongoing program to evaluate the health risks and benefits of contraception use is needed in both developing and developed countries. Such research will help scientists to understand the effects of specific methods under different conditions of use. Such studies would be especially useful in the case of oral contraceptives and other steroid or hormonal methods because the evolution of methods (e.g., changes in dosages in oral contraceptives) and long latency period of potential health problems (e.g., cancer) means that potential risks and benefits can be understood only through long-term studies. Ongoing evaluation of oral contraceptives and other methods is also needed in both developing and developed countries to provide the depth of knowledge necessary for the refinement and improvement of contraceptive methods and guidelines for their use.

REPRODUCTIVE RISKS AND CHILDREN'S HEALTH: RISKS FOR INDIVIDUAL CHILDREN

Parents can maximize the chances of survival and good health for each of their children by lengthening the intervals between births, avoiding pregnancies at very young and older ages, and avoiding higher-parity pregnancies. Firstborn children also appear to have higher risks of morbidity and mortality. However, parents obviously cannot increase their children's chances of survival by avoiding having a first birth, although they may be able to improve their firstborn's survival chances by delaying the birth until their early twenties and having their second child more than two years after their first.

The association between birth spacing and child survival has been observed in developing countries, in high-mortality historical populations, and in contemporary industrialized countries. In this wide range of historical and contemporary populations, children born after short birth intervals have higher mortality than children born after longer intervals. Furthermore, the relationship remains important in studies that hold some of the potentially confounding factors constant. However, when potentially confounding factors are held constant, it appears that the detrimental effects of older maternal age and higher birth order on children's health are less important than previously thought.

Our understanding of the mechanisms affecting the observed associations between health and birth spacing as well as for maternal age, birth order, and family size remains incomplete. While a relationship between close birth spacing and higher infant and child mortality is widely observed, we do not yet know whether this relationship is due to birthweight or gestational age or some other factor. In contemporary developing countries, families who use contraception to space their births may also be more likely to use health services when their children are ill. Until further research has been completed, caution is necessary when drawing conclusions about the amount of improvement in children's survival that may result from changes in reproductive patterns. Nonetheless, given the breadth of the available evidence—as well as the likelihood that there are important indirect benefits of lower fertility on family health and well-being—we believe that parents who wish to improve their children's chances of survival should avoid short birth intervals, births at very young and at older ages, and higher-order births. The effects of this strategy are likely to be greater where living standards are poor, the incidence of disease is high, and parents do not have access to adequate health care.

Given the strength of the observed relationship between short birth intervals and infant and child health, policy makers, health and family planning program managers, and concerned citizens in developing countries can improve children's health by encouraging both breastfeeding and contraceptive use in order to lengthen birth intervals. With this approach the beneficial effects of breastfeeding for children's health are reinforced by the contraceptive effect of breastfeeding in delaying the next birth. In many developing countries, breastfeeding has declined during the course of development, and many mothers apparently decide to discontinue breastfeeding when they adopt contraception. It also appears that some family planning programs may discourage breastfeeding for women adopting contraception out of concern about the effects of hormonal contraception on breast milk. While more research is needed on the relationship between contraceptive use and breastfeeding and, in particular, on the extent to which women substitute one for the other, programs designed to encourage both breastfeeding and contraceptive use for birth spacing are likely to have important benefits for the health of children.

Because of the clear relationship between a reduction in the number of pregnancies a woman has and reduction in her lifetime risk of dying from reproductive causes, another potential health benefit of lower fertility for children is a reduced risk of losing their mother to illness or death. Documentation of the effects of maternal mortality on the health and well-being of children in developing countries is mostly anecdotal. However, since women remain primary caretakers for children in most countries, maternal death or illness almost certainly has severe consequences for the health and survival of young children.

AGGREGATE-LEVEL EFFECTS

Reducing fertility and avoiding high-risk pregnancies are important strategies to reduce the risk of mortality and morbidity for individual women and children. Determining the implication of widespread individual changes in reproductive patterns on aggregate measures of health, such as the infant mortality rate, however, is complex and has been the subject of considerable debate (see Trussell and Pebley, 1984; Winikoff, 1983; Bongaarts, 1988; Trussell, 1988; Palloni, 1988).

There are at least two reasons to believe that a reduction in fertility will bring about an unambiguous decline in mortality rates and an improvement in the health of a population. First, maternal mortality rates, which measure the frequency of death due to reproductive causes, are likely to decline as a consequence of a fertility decline, because women will be exposed to risks associated with pregnancy less often. In other words, if fertility rates decline, there will be fewer pregnancies, and thus fewer women exposed to the risk of dying from reproductive causes each year.

Second, at a given level of funding for health care, lower fertility rates are likely to mean better health care for each pregnant woman and child because more resources per capita will be available. As a consequence of better health care, maternal and child morbidity and mortality would be expected to decline.

Measuring the impact of change in the level and pattern of childbearing for a society is complicated by the fact that mortality rates reflect in part the distribution of pregnancies and births among high-risk and low-risk groups in the population. A change in reproductive patterns is likely to change this distribution of pregnancies and births in several ways at the same time. The end result, in some populations, may be that there is relatively little change in mortality rates as a direct consequence of change in reproductive patterns, even though the rates for specific groups may decline. Insofar as these changing patterns of reproduction are associated with lower levels of fertility, they will also be associated with lower numbers of infant deaths.

As shown in Chapter 6, one of the major effects of a fertility decline is to reduce the proportion of births to high-parity women in a population and, at the same time, to increase the proportion of first births. Currently available evidence indicates that infant mortality rates are higher for first births as well as for higher-order births. Since both first births and higher-order births have elevated risks of mortality, the effect of a fertility decline, if everything else remains the same, may be small or neutral. Because the available data indicate maternal mortality ratios are higher for first pregnancies as well as for higher-order pregnancies, this argument also applies to maternal mortality ratios, which measure the average risk of death for women associated with each pregnancy in a population.

Another type of distributional change may mean that, holding everything else constant, mortality rates might actually increase somewhat during the early part of a fertility decline. The reason is that it is often women who are at relatively low risk for infant, child, or maternal mortality who first adopt contraception as a means of reducing fertility. Thus, a larger proportion of pregnancies and births would occur to women who were at higher risk in the initial period of the fertility decline than had been the case before the decline began.

The potential scope for improving health at the societal level through changes in reproductive patterns also depends on the distribution of pregnancies and births among high- and low-risk groups in a society. In South Asia and some African countries, for example, many births occur to very young women. There is, therefore, considerable potential for improving the health of women and children by delaying the onset of childbearing. The potential for improving child health through changes in patterns of birth spacing patterns is likely to be larger in Latin American countries than in other areas of the developing world because of the high proportion of short birth intervals. The current scope for improvements in child health through birth spacing is considerably more limited in South Asian and sub-Saharan African countries because short birth intervals are relatively rare. A central concern for policy makers in South Asian and sub-Saharan African countries is that birth intervals may become shorter during the course of modernization because of the decline in breastfeeding and postpartum abstinence. If such changes occur, the effect may be to slow the pace of infant and child mortality decline relative to the pace that would be achieved if longer birth spacing had been maintained.

In reality, fertility declines and changes in reproductive patterns do not occur in isolation. They are accompanied by (and brought about by) a variety of other important social and economic changes as well as by governmental policy initiatives. These changes themselves are likely to have major effects on health and mortality independent of their relation to fertility, and declines in fertility may in part be responsive to these improvements in health and mortality conditions. In fact, most countries have experienced fairly continuous mortality declines while undergoing fertility transitions, and interruptions in the mortality decline have generally been due to natural disasters, economic calamity, or major epidemics.

INDIRECT EFFECTS OF REPRODUCTIVE CHANGE ON THE HEALTH OF WOMEN AND CHILDREN

Lower fertility and changing reproductive patterns may also have important indirect effects on the health of women and children. These effects include shifting attitudes away from fatalism, making it feasible for women to develop roles independent of motherhood, and increasing the resources available for each member of the family because of smaller family sizes. These indirect effects are difficult to document, but in the long run they may be equally or more significant than the direct effects of changing reproductive patterns.

Considerable work remains before we have a clear understanding of the indirect effects of changing reproductive patterns on maternal and child health. There is particular need to understand how family structure and the process of family decision making in developing countries adjusts to changing economic, social, and demographic situations. Seemingly minor changes in one element of reproductive patterns may have long-term consequences that may improve the health and well-being of all family members. For example, Ryder (1976) argues that delaying the age at which women in developing countries have their first birth is of particular importance to these societies because it allows time for women to participate in other, nonfamilial social roles, such as that of a student or worker.

Exposure to modern medical services may also have significant long-term consequences on the attitudes of women and children beyond the immediate effects of treatment. For example, women may be more likely to continue treatment if their first exposure to modern medicine produces positive results. Increasing our understanding of how attitudes and family health care are influenced by exposure to modern health care, including family planning services, is crucial to policy makers.

FAMILY PLANNING AND THE HEALTH OF WOMEN AND CHILDREN

One aim of this report is to evaluate the potential for family planning to bring about additional improvements in the health of women and children. At several points, we have emphasized the complexity of the relationships involved, but the implications of the available evidence are clear. Maternal, infant, and child mortality and morbidity remain important problems throughout the developing world and are clearly related to reproductive patterns. Although there is a great deal of variation in the effect that reproduction has on the health of individuals, families, and countries, the reduction of high-risk pregnancies typically would have a positive impact on the health of mothers and children throughout the developing world.

Contraceptive use and controlled fertility are safer than unregulated childbearing. Unsafe abortions are a significant cause of maternal mortality in many developing countries, a finding that must be considered by countries debating the merits of making safe abortions available. Greater control of reproduction would improve maternal and child health by reducing births, especially high-parity births, and by reducing closely spaced pregnancies. Easy access to contraceptive services should be encouraged, particularly in conjunction with efforts to increase prenatal care, to improve breastfeeding practices, and to advance other health services. Efforts to increase education, especially female literacy, and to improve nutritional status may act synergistically with family planning and health services to improve maternal and child health.

It should also be clear from this report that additional research is needed in many areas before we understand adequately the causal linkages between reproduction and women's and children's health. While this research is being carried out, however, government officials, policy makers, public health practitioners, and individuals everywhere must make decisions about the best ways to improve the health of individuals and families. Family planning activities have an important potential role as a component of health programs directed toward improving the health of women and children.

References

Aaby, P., J. Bukh, I.M. Lisse, and A.J. Smits
    1984   Overcrowding and intensive exposure as determinants of measles mortality. *American Journal of Epidemiology* 120(1):49-63.

Affandi, G., S.S.I. Santoso, Djajadilaga, W. Hadisaputra, F.A. Moeloek, J. Prihartono, F. Lubis, and R.S. Samil
    1987   Pregnancy after removal of Norplant® implants contraceptive. *Contraception* 36(2):203-209.

Aitken, I.W., and B. Walls
    1986   Maternal height and cephalopelvic disproportion in Sierra Leone. *Tropical Doctor* 16(3):132-134.

Alauddin, M.
    1987   Maternal mortality in rural Bangladesh: The Tangail District. *Studies in Family Planning* 17(1):13-21.

Arkutu, A.A.
    1978   A clinical study of maternal age and parturition in 2791 Tanzanian primiparae. *International Journal of Gynaecology and Obstetrics* 16(1):20-23.

Bain C., C.H. Hennekens, F.E. Speizer, B. Rosner, W. Willett, and C. Belanger
    1982   Oral contraceptive use and malignant melanoma. *Journal of the National Cancer Institute* 68(4):537-539.

Bairagi, R.
    1986   Food crisis, nutrition, and female children in rural Bangladesh. *Population and Development Review* 12(2):307-315.

Barlow, D.
    1977   The condom and gonorrhea. *The Lancet* 2:811-812.

Bean, Lee L., Geraldine P. Mineau, and Douglas L. Anderton
    1987   Reproductive Behavior and Child Survival Among Nineteenth-Century Mormons. Paper prepared for the Working Group on the Health Consequences of Contraceptive Use and Controlled Fertility. Committee on Population, National Research Council, Washington, D.C.

Beral, V., S. Evans, H. Shaw, and G. Milton
    1984   Oral contraceptive use and malignant melanoma in Australia. *British Journal of Cancer* 50(5):681-685.

Beral, V., P. Hannaford, and C. Kay
  1988   Oral contraceptive use and malignancies of the genital tract. *The Lancet* 2:1331-1335.
Bhatia, J.C.
  1985   Maternal Mortality in Anantapur District, India: Preliminary Findings of a Study. WHO
         FHE/PMM/85.9.16. WHO Interregional Meeting on Prevention of Maternal Mortality,
         Geneva, 11-15 November.
Bhatia, S., S. Becker, and Y.J. Kim
  1987   The effect of oral contraceptive acceptance on fertility in the postpartum period. *Interna-
         tional Journal of Gynaecology and Obstetrics* 25(Suppl):1-11.
Bhiwandiwala, P.P., S.D. Mumford, and P.J. Feldblum
  1983   Menstrual pattern changes following laparoscopic sterilization with different occlusion
         techniques: A review of 10,004 cases. *American Journal of Obstetrics and Gynecology*
         145(6):684-694.
Bijur, P., J. Golding, and M. Kurzon
  1988   Childhood accidents, family size, and birth order. *Social Science and Medicine* 26(8):839-
         843.
Boerma, J.T., and H.A.W. van Vianen
  1984   Birth interval, mortality and growth of children in a rural area of Kenya. *Journal of
         Biosocial Science* 16(4):475-486.
Bongaarts, J.
  1987   Does family planning reduce infant mortality rates? *Population and Development Review*
         13(2):323-334.
  1988   Does family planning reduce infant mortality rates?: Reply. *Population and Development
         Review* 14(1):188-190.
Boston Collaborative Drug Surveillance Program
  1974   Surgically confirmed gallbladder disease, versus thromboembolism, and breast tumors in
         relation to postmenopausal estrogen therapy. *New England Journal of Medicine* 2(290):15-
         19.
Bray, R.S., and M.J. Anderson
  1979   Falciparum malaria and pregnancy. *Transactions of the Royal Society of Medicine and
         Hygiene* 73:427-431.
Brinton, L.A., G.R. Huggins, H.F. Lehman, K. Mallin, D.A. Savitz, E. Trapido, J. Rosenthal, and R.
         Hoover
  1986   Long-term use of oral contraceptives and risk of invasive cervical cancer. *International
         Journal of Cancer* 38(3):339-344.
Brinton, L.A., M.P. Vessey, R. Flavel, and D. Yeates
  1981   Risk factors for benign breast disease. *American Journal of Epidemiology* 113(3):203-
         214.
Cantrelle, P., and H. Leridon
  1971   Breastfeeding, mortality in childhood and fertility in a rural zone of Senegal. *Population
         Studies* 25(3):505-533.
Casterline, J.B., and J. Trussell
  1980   *Age at First Birth*. World Fertility Survey Comparative Studies No. 15. Voorburg,
         Netherlands: International Statistical Institute.
Celentano, D.D., A.C. Klassen, C.S. Weissman, and B. Rosenstein
  1987   The role of contraceptive use in cervical cancer: The Maryland cervical cancer case-
         control study. *American Journal of Epidemiology* 126(4):592-604.
Centers for Disease Control
  1987   Antibody to human immunodeficiency virus in female prostitutes. *Morbidity and Mortal-
         ity Weekly Report* 36(11):157-161.
  1988   Condoms for prevention of sexually transmitted diseases. *Morbidity and Mortality
         Weekly Report* 37(9):133-137.
Centers for Disease Control and the National Institute of Child Health and Human Development
         (Cancer and Steroid Hormone Study)
  1986   Oral-contraceptive use and the risk of breast cancer. *The New England Journal of
         Medicine* 315(7):405-411.
  1987a Combination oral contraceptive use and the risk of endometrial cancer. *The Journal of the
         American Medical Association* 257(6):796-800.

1987b The reduction in risk of ovarian cancer associated with oral-contraceptive use. *The New England Journal of Medicine* 316(11):650-655.

Chen, L.C., M.C. Gesche, S. Ahmed, A.I. Chowdhury, and W.H. Mosley
  1975 Maternal mortality in Bangladesh. *Studies in Family Planning* 5(11):334-341.

Chen, L.C., E. Huq, and S. D'Souza
  1981 Sex bias in the family allocation of food and health care in rural Bangladesh. *Population and Development Review* 7(1):55-70.

Chi, I.C., T. Agoestina, and J. Harbin
  1981 Maternal mortality at twelve teaching hospitals in Indonesia— An epidemiologic analysis. *International Journal of Gynaecology and Obstetrics* 19(4):259-266.

Chow, W.H., J.R. Daling, N.S. Weiss, D.E. Moore, and R. Soderstrom
  1985 Vaginal douching as a potential risk factor for tubal ectopic pregnancies. *American Journal of Obstetrics and Gynecology* 153(7):727-729.

Clark, Carol A.M.
  1981 Demographic and Socioeconomic Correlates of Infant Growth in Guatemala. Paper presented at the annual meeting of the Population Association of America, March 26-28.

Cleland, J.G., and S. Rutstein
  1986 Contraception and birthspacing. *International Family Planning Perspectives* 12(3):83-90.

Cleland, J.G., and Z.A. Sathar
  1984 The effect of birthspacing on childhood mortality in Pakistan. *Population Studies* 38(3):401-418.

Coale, A., and D.R. McNeil
  1972 The distribution by age of the frequency of first marriage in a female cohort. *Journal of the American Statistical Association* 67:743-749.

Conant, M., D. Hardy, J. Sematinger, D. Spicer, and J.A. Levy
  1986 Condoms prevent transmission of AIDS-associated retrovirus. *The Journal of the American Medical Association* 255(13):1706.

Conant, M.A., D.W. Spicer, and C.D. Smith
  1984 Herpes simplex virus transmission: Condom studies. *Sexually Transmitted Diseases* 11(2):94-95.

Costello, C.
  1986 Maternal and Child Health in Rural Uganda: The Role of Nutrition. PhD dissertation, University of Pennsylvania.

Cowan, M.E., and G.E. Cree
  1973 A note on the susceptibility of N. gonorrhoeae to contraceptive agent Nonyl-P. *British Journal of Venereal Diseases* 49(1):65-66.

Cramer, D.W., M.B. Goldman, I. Schiff, S. Belisle, B. Albrecht, B. Stadel, M. Gibson, E. Wilson, R. Stillman, and I. Thompson
  1987 The relationship of tubal infertility to barrier method and oral contraceptive use. *The Journal of the American Medical Association* 257(18):2446-2450.

Cramer, D.W., I. Schiff, S.C. Schoenbaum, M. Gibson, S. Belisle, B. Albrecht, R.J. Stillman, M.J. Berger, E. Wilson, B.V. Stadel, and M. Seibel
  1985 Tubal infertility and the intrauterine device. *New England Journal of Medicine* 312(15):941-947.

Daling, J.R., N.S. Weiss, B.J. Metch, W.H. Chow, R.M. Soderstrom, D.E. Moore, L.R. Spadoni, and B.V. Stadel
  1985 Primary tubal infertility in relation to the use of an intrauterine device. *New England Journal of Medicine* 312(15):937-941.

Das Gupta, M.
  1987 Selective discrimination against female children in rural Punjab. *Population and Development Review* 13(1):77-100.

DaVanzo, Julie, W.P. Butz, and J.-P. Habicht
  1983 How biological and behavioral influences on mortality in Malaysia vary during the first year of life. *Population Studies* 37(3):381-402.

DaVanzo, Julie, J.-P. Habicht, and W.P. Butz
  1984 Assessing socioeconomic correlates of birthweight in peninsular Malaysia: Ethnic differences and changes over time. *Social Science and Medicine* 18(5):387-404.

DaVanzo, Julie, and E.H. Starbird
    1989   Correlates of Short Inter-Birth Intervals in Malaysia: The Roles of Breastfeeding and Contraceptive Use. Paper presented at meeting of the Population Association of America, Baltimore, Maryland, March.

David, Henry P., Z. Dytrych, Z. Matejcek, and V. Schueller
    1988   *Born Unwanted: Developmental Effects of Denied Abortion.* New York: Springer Publishing Co.

Diaz, S., M. Pavez, P. Miranda, E.D.B. Johansson, and H.B. Croxatto
    1987   Long-term follow-up of women treated with Norplant® implants. *Contraception* 35(6):551-567.

Dixon-Mueller, Ruth
    1989   Psychosocial consequences to women of contraceptive use and controlled fertility. In A.M. Parnell (ed.), *Contraceptive Use and Controlled Fertility: Health Issues for Women and Children.* Washington, D.C.: National Academy Press.

Donaldson, P.J., and D.J. Nichols
    1978   The changing tempo of fertility in Korea. *Population Studies* 32(July):231-249.

Doyle, P., D. Morley, M. Woodland, and J. Cole
    1978   Birth intervals, survival and growth in a Nigerian village. *Journal of Biosocial Science* 10(1):81-94.

D'Souza, S., and L.C. Chen
    1980   Sex differentials in mortality in rural Bangladesh. *Population and Development Review* 6(2):257-270.

Ebeling, K., P. Nischan, and Ch. Schindler
    1987   Use of oral contraceptives and risk of invasive cervical cancer in previously screened women. *International Journal of Cancer* 39(4):427-430.

Efiong, E.I., and M.O. Banjoko
    1975   The obstetric performance of Nigerian primigravidae aged 16 and under. *British Journal of Obstetrics and Gynaecology* 82(3):228-233.

Erickson, J.D., and T. Bjerkedal
    1978   Interpregnancy interval: Association with birth weight, stillbirth, and neonatal death. *Journal of Epidemiology and Community Health* 32(2):124-130.

Faundes, A., B. Fanjul, G. Henriquez, G. Mora, and C. Tognola
    1974   Influencia de la edad y de la paridad sobre algunos parametros de morbilidad materna y sobre la morbimortalidad fetal. *Revista Chilena de Obstetrica y Ginecologia* 37(1):6-14.

Fedrick, J., and P. Adelstein
    1973   Influence of pregnancy spacing on outcome of pregnancy. *British Medical Journal* 4:753-756.

Feldblum, P.J., and J.A. Fortney
    1988   Condoms, spermicides, and the transmission of human immunodeficiency virus: A review of the literature. *American Journal of Public Health* 78(1):52-54.

Ferraz, E.M., R.H. Gray, P.L. Fleming, and T.M. Maria
    1988   Interpregnancy interval and low birthweight: Findings from a case-control study. *American Journal of Epidemiology* 128:1111-1116.

Fihn, S.D., R.H. Latham, P. Roberts, K. Running, and W.E. Stamm
    1985   Association between diaphragm use and urinary tract infection. *The Journal of the American Medical Association* 254(2):240-245.

Fischl, M.A., G.M. Dickinson, G.B. Scott, N. Kilmas, M.A. Fletcher, and W. Parks
    1987   Evaluation of heterosexual partners, children, and household contacts of adults with AIDS. *The Journal of the American Medical Association* 257(5):640-644.

Fleming, P.L., and R.H. Gray
    1988a   Child Growth in Relation to the Succeeding Birth Interval. Unpublished manuscript. Department of Population Dynamics, Johns Hopkins University.
    1988b   Some Effects of the Preceding Birth Interval on Birth Weight and Subsequent Growth. Unpublished manuscript. Department of Population Dynamics, Johns Hopkins University.

Forman, D., T.J. Vincent, and R. Doll
    1986   Cancer of the liver and the use of oral contraceptives. *British Medical Journal* 292:1357-1361.

Fortney, J.A., and J.E. Higgins
  1984   The effect of birth intervals on perinatal survival and birth weight. *Public Health* 98(2):73-83.
Fortney, J.A., J.E. Higgins, K.I. Kennedy, L.E. Laufe, and L. Wilkens
  1986   Delivery and neonatal mortality among 10,749 breeches. *American Journal of Public Health* 76:982-985.
Fortney, J.A., I. Susanti, S. Gadalla, S. Saleh, P.J. Feldblum, and M. Potts
  1985   Maternal Mortality in Indonesia and Egypt. WHO FHE/PMM/85.9.13. WHO Interregional Meeting on Prevention of Maternal Mortality, Geneva, 11-15 November.
Foster, Andrew D., Alauddin Chowdhury, Jane Menken, and Sandra L. Huffman
  1986   Age at Menarche and its Influence on Fertility. Fertility Determinants Research Note No. 10. The Population Council, New York.
Foster, S.O.
  1984   Immunizable and respiratory diseases and child mortality. *Population and Development Review* 10(Suppl.):119-140.
Foxman, B., and R.R. Frerichs
  1985   Epidemiology of urinary tract infection: Diaphragm use and sexual intercourse. *American Journal of Public Health* 75(11):1308-1313.
Geronimus, A.T.
  1987   On teenage childbearing and neonatal mortality in the United States. *Population and Development Review* 13(2):245-279.
Goldacre, M.J., J.A. Clarke, M.A. Heasman, and M.P. Vessey
  1978   Followup of vasectomy using medical record linkage. *American Journal of Epidemiology* 108(3):176-180.
Goldacre, M.J., M. Vessey, J. Clarke, and M. Heasman
  1979   Record linkage study of morbidity following vasectomy. Pp. 567-569 in I.H. Lepow and R. Crozier (eds.), *Vasectomy: Immunologic and Pathophysiologic Effects in Animals and Man.* New York: Academic Press.
Goldman, N., S.O. Rutstein, and S. Singh
  1985   *Assessment of the Quality of Data in 41 WFS Surveys: A Comparative Approach.* World Fertility Survey Comparative Studies No. 44. Voorburg, Netherlands: International Statistical Institute.
Gomez de Leon, Jose, and J.E. Potter
  1989   Modelling the inverse association between breastfeeding and contraceptive use. *Population Studies* 43 (March/1):69-93.
Gray, R.H.
  1984   A case-control study of ectopic pregnancy in developed and developing countries. Pp. 354-364 in G.I. Zatuchni, A. Goldsmith, and J.J. Sciarra (eds.), *Intrauterine Contraception: Advances and Future Prospects.* Philadelphia: Harper and Row.
  1985   Reduced risk of pelvic inflammatory disease with injectable contraceptives. *The Lancet* 1:1046.
Gray, R.H., and O.M. Campbell
  1985   Epidemiologic trends of PID in contraceptive use. In G.I. Zatuchni, A. Goldsmith, and J.S. Sciarra (eds.), *Intrauterine Contraception: Advances and Future Prospects.* Philadelphia: Harper and Row.
Greenwood, A.M., B.M. Greenwood, A.K. Bradley, K. Williams, F.C. Shenton, S. Tulloch, P. Byass, and F.S.J. Oldfield
  1987   A prospective survey of the outcome of pregnancy in a rural area in the Gambia. *Bulletin of the World Health Organization* 65(5):635-643.
Grimes, D.A.
  1987   Intrauterine devices and pelvic inflammatory disease: Recent developments. *Contraception* 36(1):97-109.
Grimes, D.A., A.P. Satterthwaite, R.W. Rochat, and N. Akhter
  1982   Deaths from contraceptive sterilization in Bangladesh: Rates, causes, and prevention. *Obstetrics and Gynecology* 60(5):635-640.
Grossman, Michael, and Steven Jacobowitz
  1981   Variations in infant mortality rates among counties of the United States: The roles of public policies and programs. *Demography* 18(4):695-713.

Gubhaju, B.
  1986   Effect of birth spacing on infant and child mortality in rural Nepal. *Journal of Biosocial Science* 18(4):435-447.
Haaga, John
  1989   Mechanisms for the Association of Maternal Age, Parity, and Birth Spacing with Infant Health. In A.M. Parnell (ed.), *Contraceptive Use and Controlled Fertility: Health Issues for Women and Children*. Washington, D.C.: National Academy Press.
Habicht, J.-P., J. DaVanzo, W.P. Butz, and L. Meyers
  1985   The contraceptive role of breastfeeding. *Population Studies* 39:213-232.
Hansen, J.P.
  1986   Older maternal age and pregnancy outcome: A review of the literature. *Obstetrical and Gynecological Survey* 41:726-742.
Harris, R.W.C., L.A. Brinton, R.H. Cowdell, D.C.G. Skegg, P.G. Smith, M.P. Vessey, and R. Doll
  1980   Characteristics of women with dysplasia or carcinoma *in situ* of the cervix uteri. *British Journal of Cancer* 42(3):359-369.
Harrison, K.A., and L.A. Rossiter
  1985   Child-bearing, health and social priorities: A survey of 22,774 consecutive hospital births in Zaria, Northern Nigeria. *British Journal of Obstetrics and Gynaecology* (Supplement 5)(92):1-119.
Hart, G.
  1974   Factors influencing venereal infection in a war environment. *British Journal of Venereal Diseases* 50(1):68-72.
Hatcher, R.A., F. Guest, F. Stewart, G.K. Stewart, J. Trussell, S.C. Bowen, and W. Cates
  1988   *Contraceptive Technology 1988-1989*. New York: Irvington Publishers, Inc.
Heartwell, S.F., and S. Schlesselman
  1983   Risk of uterine perforation among users of intrauterine devices. *Obstetrics and Gynecology* 61(1):31-36.
Henderson, B.E., S. Preston-Martin, H.A. Edmondson, R.L. Peters, and M.C. Pike
  1983   Hepatocellular carcinoma and oral contraceptives. *British Journal of Cancer* 48(3):437-440.
Henshaw, Stanley K.
  1986   Induced abortion: A worldwide perspective. *Family Planning Perspectives* 18(6):250-254.
Hicks, D.R., L.S. Martin, J.P. Getchell, J.L. Heath, D.P. Francis, J.S. McDougal, J.W. Curran, and B. Voeller
  1985   Inactivation of HTLV-III/LAV-infected cultures of normal human lymphocytes by Nonoxynol-9 in vitro. *The Lancet* 2:1422-1423.
Hobcraft, J.
  1987   Does Family Planning Save Children's Lives? Paper prepared for the International Conference on Better Health for Women and Children through Family Planning, Nairobi, October 5-9.
Hobcraft, J.N., J.W. McDonald, and S.O. Rutstein
  1985   Demographic determinants of infant and early child mortality: A comparative analysis. *Population Studies* 39(3):363-385.
Holly, E.A., N.S. Weiss, and J.M. Liff
  1983   Cutaneous melanoma in relation to exogenous hormones and reproductive factors. *Journal of the National Cancer Institute* 70(5):827-831.
Honda, G.D., L. Bernstein, R.K. Ross, S. Greenland, V. Gerkins, and B.E. Henderson
  1988   Vasectomy, cigarette smoking, and age at first sexual intercourse as risk factors for prostate cancer in middle-aged men. *British Journal of Cancer* 57(3):326-331.
Hook, E.B.
  1985   Maternal age, paternal age, and human chromosome abnormality: Nature, magnitude, etiology, and mechanism of effects. *Basic Life Sciences* 36.
Hooper, R.R., G.H. Reynolds, O.G. Jones, A. Zaidi, P.J. Wiesner, K.P. Latimer, A. Lester, A.F. Campbell, W.O. Harrison, W.W. Karney, and K.K. Holmes
  1978   Cohort study of venereal disease. I. The risk of gonorrhea transmission from infected women to men. *American Journal of Epidemiology* 108(2):136-144.

Horsburgh, C.R., Jr., J.M. Douglas, and F.M. LaForce
  1987   Preventive strategies in sexually transmitted diseases for the primary care physician. *The Journal of the American Medical Association* 258(6):815-821.

Institute of Medicine
  1973   *Infant Death: An Analysis by Maternal Risks and Health Care*, Vol. 1. Washington, D.C.: National Academy of Sciences.
  1985   *Preventing Low Birthweight.* Washington, D.C.: National Academy Press.

Irwin, K.L., L. Rosero-Bixby, M.W. Oberle, N.C. Lee, A.S. Whatley, J.A. Fortney, and M.G. Bonhomme
  1988   Oral contraceptives and cervical cancer risk in Costa Rica: Detection bias or causal association? *The Journal of the American Medical Association* 259(1):59-64.

Jelley, D., and R.J. Madeley
  1983   Antenatal care in Maputo, Mozambique. *Journal of Epidemiology and Community Health* 37(2):111-116.

Jelliffe, D.B.
  1976   Maternal nutrition and lactation. In *CIBA Foundation Symposium: Breastfeeding and the Mother.* Amsterdam: Excerpta Medica.

Jick, H., M.T. Hannan, A. Stergachis, F. Heidrich, D.R. Perera, and K.J. Rothman
  1982   Vaginal spermicides and gonorrhea. *The Journal of the American Medical Association* 248(13):1619-1621.

Judson, F.N., J.M. Enret, G.M. Bodin, M.J. Levin, and C.A.M. Rietmeijer
In press   In vitro evaluations of condoms with and without Nonoynol-9 as physical and chemical barriers against chlamydia trachomatis, herpes simplex virus type 2, and human immunodeficiency virus. *Sexually Transmitted Diseases* (Supplement).

Kambic, R., R.H. Gray, and J.L. Simpson
  1988   Outcome of Pregnancy in NFP Users. Institute for International Studies in Natural Family Planning, Georgetown University.

Katznelson, S., W.L. Drew, and L. Mintz
  1984   Efficacy of the condom as a barrier to the transmission of cytomegalovirus. *Journal of Infectious Diseases* 150(1):155-157.

Kelaghan, J., G.L. Rubin, H.W. Ory, and P.M. Layde
  1982   Barrier-method contraceptives and pelvic inflammatory disease. *The Journal of the American Medical Association* 248(2):184-187.

Khan, A.R., F.A. Jahan, and S.F. Begum
  1986   Maternal mortality in rural Bangladesh: The Jamalpur District. *Studies in Family Planning* 17(1):7-12.

Klebanoff, M.A.
  1988   Short interpregnancy interval and the risk of low birthweight. *American Journal of Public Health* 78(6):667-670.

Knodel, J., and A.I. Hermalin
  1984   Effects of birth rank, maternal age, birth interval, and sibship size on infant and child mortality: Evidence from 18th and 19th century reproductive histories. *American Journal of Public Health* 74(10):1098-1106.

Koenig, M.A., V. Fauveau, A.I. Chowdhury, J. Chakraborty, and M.A. Khan
  1988a Maternal mortality in Matlab, Bangladesh: 1976-85. *Studies in Family Planning* 19(2):69-80.

Koenig, M.A., J. Phillips, O. Campbell, and S. D'Souza
  1988b Birth Intervals and Childhood Mortality in Rural Bangladesh. Unpublished manuscript. The Population Council, New York.

Kramer, M.S.
  1987   Intrauterine growth and gestational age determinants. *Pediatrics* 80:502-511.

Kronmal, R.A., E. Alderman, J.N. Krieger, T. Killip, J.W. Kennedy, and M.W. Athearn
  1988   Vasectomy and urolithiasis. *The Lancet* 1:22-23.

Kwast, Barbara E., R.W. Rochat, and W. Kidane-Mariam
  1986   Maternal mortality in Addis Ababa, Ethiopia. *Studies in Family Planning* 17(6):288-301.

Kwast, B.E., and J.A. Stevens
  1987   Viral hepatitis as a major cause of maternal mortality in Addis Ababa, Ethiopia. *International Journal of Gynaecology and Obstetrics* 25(2):99-106.

Layde, P.M., M.P. Vessey, and D. Yeates
    1982   Risk factors for gall-bladder disease: A cohort study of young women attending family planning clinics. *Journal of Epidemiology and Community Health* 36(4):274-278.
Lee, N.C., G.L. Rubin, and R. Borucki
    1988   The intrauterine device and pelvic inflammatory disease revisited: New results from the Women's Health Study. *Obstetrics and Gynecology* 72(1):1-6.
Lee, Nancy C., Herbert B. Peterson, and Susan Y. Chu
    1989   Health effects of contraception. In A.M. Parnell (ed.), *Contraceptive Use and Controlled Fertility: Health Issues for Women and Children*. Washington, D.C.: National Academy Press.
Lettenmaier, C., L. Liskin, C. Church, and J. Harris
    1988   Mothers' lives matter: Maternal health in the community. *Population Reports* Series L, No. 7. Population Information Program, Johns Hopkins University.
Lindpainter, L.S., N. Jahan, A.P. Satterthwaite, and S. Zimicki
    1982   Maternity-Related Mortality in Matlab Thana, Bangladesh. Unpublished manuscript. International Centre for Diarrheal Disease Research, Bangladesh.
Liskin, L.S., R. Blackburn, and R. Ghani
    1987   Hormonal contraception: New long-acting methods. *Population Reports* Series K, No. 3.
Liskin, L.S., and W.F. Quillin
    1982   Long-acting progestins: Promise and prospects. *Population Reports* Series K, No. 2.
London, K.A., J. Cushing, S.O. Rutstein, J. Cleland, J.E. Anderson, L. Morris and S.H. Moore
    1985   Fertility and family planning surveys: An update. *Population Reports* Series M, No. 8.
Lunt, R.
    1984   Worldwide early detection of cervical cancer. *Obstetrics and Gynecology* 63(5):708-713.
Lynch, K.A.
    1987   Maternal Mortality in the European Past. Paper prepared for the Working Group on the Health Consequences of Contraceptive Use and Controlled Fertility. Committee on Population, National Research Council, Washington, D.C.
McAnarney, E.R.
    1987   Young maternal age and adverse neonatal outcome. *American Journal of Diseases of Children* 141(1):1053-1059.
McDonald, P.
    1984   *Nuptiality and Completed Fertility: A Study of Starting, Stopping and Spacing Behavior.* World Fertility Survey Comparative Studies No. 35. Voorburg, Netherlands: International Statistical Institute.
McGregor, I.A.
    1984   Epidemiology, malaria and pregnancy. *American Journal of Tropical Medicine and Hygiene* 33:517-525.
McGregor, I.A., M.E. Wilson, and W.Z. Billewicz
    1983   Malaria infection of the placenta in The Gambia, West Africa; its incidence and relationship to stillbirth, birthweight and placental weight. *Transactions of the Royal Society of Tropical Medicine and Hygiene* 77(2):232-244.
McNeilly, A.S.
    1977   Physiology of lactation. *Journal of Biosocial Science* Supplement(4):5-21.
McPherson, K., A. Neil, M.P. Vessey, and R. Doll
    1983   Oral contraceptives and breast cancer. *The Lancet* 2:1414-1415.
Massey, F.J., Jr., G.S. Bernstein, W.M. O'Fallon, L.M. Schuman, A.H. Coulson, R. Crozier, J.S. Mandel, R.B. Benjamin, et al.
    1984   Vasectomy and health: Results from a large cohort study. *The Journal of the American Medical Association* 252(8):1023-1029.
Meirik, O., E. Lund, H.-O. Adami, R. Bergström, T. Christofferson, P. Bergsjö
    1986   Oral contraceptive use and breast cancer in young women. *The Lancet* 2:650-654.
Merchant K., and R. Martorell
    1988   Frequent reproductive cycling: Does it lead to nutritional depletion of mothers? *Progress in Food and Nutrition* 12:339-369.
Mhango C., R. Rochat, and A. Arkutu
    1986   Reproductive mortality in Lusaka, Zambia, 1982-1983. *Studies In Family Planning* 17(5):243-256.

Miller, Jane E.
1989   Is the relationship between birth intervals and perinatal mortality spurious? Evidence from Hungary and Sweden. *Population Studies* 43:forthcoming.
Millman, S.
1985   Breastfeeding and contraception: Why the inverse association? *Studies in Family Planning* 16(2):61-75.
1986   Trends in breastfeeding in a dozen developing countries. *International Family Planning Perspectives* 12(3):91-95.
Morrow, R.H., Jr., H.F. Smetana, F.T. Sai, and J.H. Edgcomb
1968   Unusual features of viral hepatitis in Accra, Ghana. *Annals of Internal Medicine* 68(6):1250-1264.
Neuberger, J., D. Forman, R. Doll, and R. Williams
1986   Oral contraceptives and hepatocellular carcinoma. *British Medical Journal* 292:1355-1357.
Niswander, K.R., and M. Gordon
1972   *The Women and Their Pregnancies: The Collaborative Perinatal Study of the National Institute of Neurological Diseases and Stroke.* Washington, D.C.: U.S. Government Printing Office.
Omran, A.R., and C.C. Standley (eds.)
1981   *Further Studies on Family Formation Patterns and Health.* Geneva: World Health Organization.
Ory, H.W., J.D. Forrest, and R. Lincoln
1983   *Making Choices: Evaluating the Health Risks and Benefits of Birth Control Methods.* New York: The Alan Guttmacher Institute.
Ory, H.W., and the Women's Health Study
1981   Ectopic pregnancy and intrauterine contraceptive devices: New perspectives. *Obstetrics and Gynecology* 57(2):137-144.
Overall, J.C.
1987   Viral infections of the fetus and neonate. Pp. 966-1007 in R.D. Feigin and J.D. Cherry (eds.), *Textbook of Pediatric Infectious Diseases*, 2nd ed. Philadelphia: W.B. Saunders.
Palloni, A.
1985   Health conditions in Latin America and policies for mortality changes. In Jacques Vallin and Alan Lopez (eds.), *Health Policy, Social Policy, and Mortality Prospects.* Proceedings of a seminar, Paris, February 28-March 4, 1983. Liege: Ordina Editions.
1988   On the role of crises in historical perspective: An exchange. *Population and Development Review* 14(1):145-158.
Palloni, A., and S. Millman
1986   Effects of inter-birth intervals and breastfeeding on infant and early childhood mortality. *Population Studies* 40(2):215-236.
Pardthaisong, T., R.H. Gray, and E.B. McDaniel
1980   Return of fertility after discontinuation of depot-medroxyprogesterone acetate and intra-uterine devices in Northern Thailand. *The Lancet* 1:509-512.
Pebley, Anne R., and Julie DaVanzo
1988   Maternal Depletion and Child Survival in Guatemala and Malaysia. Paper presented at meeting of the Population Association of America, New Orleans, April.
Pebley, Anne R., Howard I. Goldberg, and Jane Menken
1985   Contraceptive use during lactation in developing countries. *Studies in Family Planning* 16(1):40-51.
Pebley, Anne, John Knodel, and Albert I. Hermalin
1988   The Influence of Reproductive Patterns on Infant Mortality: Evidence from Family Reconstitution Data for 18th and 19th Century German Villages. Paper presented at the 13th annual meeting of the Social Science History Association, Chicago, November 3-6.
Pebley, A.R., and S. Millman
1986   Birthspacing and child survival. *International Family Planning Perspectives* 12(3):71-79.
Pebley, A.R., and P.W. Stupp
1987   Reproductive patterns and child mortality in Guatemala. *Demography* 24(1):43-60.

Perrin, E.B., J.S. Woods, T. Namekata, J. Yagi, R.A. Bruce, and V. Hofer
  1984   Long-term effect of vasectomy on coronary heart disease. *American Journal of Public Health* 74(2):128-132.
Peterson, H.B., F. DeStefano, G.L. Rubin, J.R. Greenspan, N.C. Lee, and H.W. Ory
  1982   Mortality risk associated with tubal sterilization in United States hospitals. *American Journal of Obstetrics and Gynecology* 143(2):125-129.
  1983   Deaths attributable to tubal sterilization in the United States, 1977-1981. *American Journal of Obstetrics and Gynecology* 146(2):131-136.
Petitti, D.B., R. Klein, H. Kipp, W. Kahn, A.B. Siegelaub, and G.D. Friedman
  1982   A survey of personal habits, symptoms of illness, and histories of disease in men with and without vasectomies. *American Journal of Public Health* 72(5):476-480.
Pike, M.C., B.E. Henderson, M.D. Krailo, A. Duke, and S. Roy
  1983   Breast cancer in young women and the use of oral contraceptives: Possible modifying effect of formulation and age at use. *The Lancet* 2:926-930.
Piper, J.M.
  1985   Oral contraceptives and cervical cancer. *Gynecologic Oncology* 22(1):1-14.
Potter, Joseph E.
  1988   Does family planning reduce infant mortality? *Population and Development Review* 14(1):179-187.
Prentice, R.L., and D.B. Thomas
  1987   On the epidemiology of oral contraceptives and disease. *Advances in Cancer Research* 49:285-401.
Puffer, R.R., and C.V. Serrano
  1973   *Patterns of Mortality in Childhood: Report of the Inter-American Investigation of Mortality in Childhood.* Washington, D.C.: Pan American Health Organization.
Ramcharan, S., F.A. Pellegrin, R.M. Ray, and J. Hsu
  1981   *The Walnut Creek Contraceptive Drug Study: A Prospective Study of the Side Effects of Oral Contraceptives,* Vol. III. Washington, D.C.: U.S. Government Printing Office.
Richard, Barbara W., and Louis Lasagne
  1987   Drug regulation in the United States and the United Kingdom: The Depo-Provera story. *Annals of Internal Medicine* 106:886-891.
Rinehart, Ward, and Adrienne Kols
  1984   Healthier mothers and children through family planning. *Population Reports* Series T, No. 27, pp. 657-696.
Rodriguez, G., and J. Trussell
  1980   Maximum Likelihood Estimation of the Parameters of Coale's Model Nuptiality Schedule. World Fertility Survey. Technical bulletin no. 7. International Statistical Institutes, Voorburg.
Rogers, S.M.
  1988   Abortion and Contraception. Paper prepared for the Working Group on the Health Consequences of Contraceptive Use and Controlled Fertility. Committee on Population, National Research Council, Washington, D.C.
Rooks, J.B., H.W. Ory, K.G. Ishak, L.T. Strauss, J.R. Greenspan, A.P. Hill, C.W. Tyler, Jr., and the Cooperative Liver Tumor Study Group
  1979   Epidemiology of hepatocellular adenoma: The role of oral contraceptive use. *The Journal of the American Medical Association* 242(7):644-648.
Rosenberg, M.J., P.J. Feldblum, W. Rojanapithayakorn, and W. Sawasdivorn
  1987   The contraceptive sponge's protection against Chlamydia trachomatis and Neisseria gonorrhoeae. *Sexually Transmitted Diseases* 14(3):147-152.
Rosenzweig, M.R., and T.P. Schultz
  1983   Estimating a household production function: Heterogeneity, the demand for health inputs, and their effects on birth weight. *Journal of Political Economy* 91(5):723-746.
Ross, J.A., S. Hong, and D.H. Huber
  1985   *Voluntary Sterilization: An International Fact Book.* New York: Association of Voluntary Sterilization, Inc.
Ross, J.A., and D.H. Huber
  1983   Acceptance and prevalence of vasectomy in developing countries. *Studies in Family Planning* 14(3):67-72.

Ross, R.K., M.C. Pike, M.P. Vessey, D. Bull, D. Yeates, and J.T. Casagrande
   1986   Risk factors for uterine fibroids: Reduced risk associated with oral contraceptives. *British Medical Journal* 293:359-362.

Royal College of General Practitioners
   1970   *Oral Contraceptives and Health.* London: Pitman Medical.
   1982   Oral contraceptives and gallbladder disease. *The Lancet* 2:957-959.

Rubin, G.L., H.W. Ory, and P.M. Layde
   1982   Oral contraceptives and pelvic inflammatory disease. *American Journal of Obstetrics and Gynecology* 144(6):630-635.

Rutstein, S.O.
   1983   *Infant and Child Mortality: Levels, Trends and Demographic Differentials.* World Fertility Survey Comparative Studies No. 24. Voorburg, Netherlands: International Statistical Institute.

Ryder, Norman B.
   1976   *Some Sociological Suggestions Concerning the Reduction of Fertility in Developing Countries.* Paper no. 37. Honolulu: East-West Population Institute.

Salah, M., A.M. Ahmed, M. Abo-Eloyoun, and M.M. Shaaban
   1987   Five-year experience with Norplant® implants in Assiut, Egypt. *Contraception* 35(6):305-316.

Schlesselman, J.J., B.V. Stadel, P. Murray, and S. Lai
   1988   Breast cancer in relation to early use of oral contraceptives: No evidence of a latent effect. *Journal of the American Medical Association* 259(12):1828-1833.

Schultz, T. Paul
   1984   Studying the impact of household economic and community variables on child mortality. *Population and Development Review* 10(Suppl.):215-235.

Schwartz, B., S. Gaventa, C.V. Broome, A. Reingold, A.W. Hightower, J.A. Perlam, P.H. Wolf, and the Toxic Shock Syndrome Study Group
   1989   Nonmenstrual toxic shock syndrome association, with barrier contraceptives: Report of a case-control study. *Review of Infectious Diseases* 2(Suppl 1):543-549.

Scrimshaw, Susan
   1978   Infant mortality and behavior in the regulation of family size. *Population Development Review* 4:383-404.

Segal, Sheldon J.
   1988   Contraceptive Innovations: Needs and Opportunities. Paper presented at Conference on Demographic and Programmatic Consequences of Contraceptive Innovations, sponsored by the Committee on Population. National Academy of Sciences, Washington, D.C., October 6-7.

Sidney, Stephen
   1987   Vasectomy and the risk of prostatic cancer and benign prostatic hypertrophy. *Journal of Urology* 138(4):795-797.

Simmons, George B., Celeste Smucker, S. Berstein, and Eric Jensen
   1982   Post-neonatal mortality in rural India: Implications of an economic model. *Demography* 19(3):371-389.

Simpson, J.L.
   1985   Relationship between congenital anomalies and contraception. *Advances in Contraception* 1(1):3-30.

Singh B., J.C. Cutler, and H.M.D. Utidjian
   1972   Studies on the development of a vaginal preparation providing both prophylaxis against venereal disease and other genital infections and contraception: II. Effect in vitro of vaginal contraceptive and noncontraceptive preparations on Treponema pallidum and Neisseria gonorrhoeae. *British Journal of Venereal Diseases* 48(3):57-64.

Singh, B., B. Postic, and J.C. Cutler
   1976   Virucidal effect of certain chemical contraceptives on Type 2 herpesvirus. *American Journal of Obstetrics and Gynecology* 126(4):422-425.

Singh, S., and B. Ferry
   1984   *Biological and Traditional Factors that Influence Fertility: Results from WFS Surveys.* World Fertility Survey Comparative Studies No. 40. Voorburg, Netherlands: International Statistical Institute.

Sivard, R.L.
    1985   *Women: A World Survey.* Washington, D.C.: World Priorities.
Sivin, I., S. Diaz, P. Holma, F. Alvarez-Sanchez, and D.N. Robertson
    1983   A four-year clinical study of Norplant® implants. *Studies in Family Planning* 14(6/7):184-191.
Smith, D.P.
    1980   *Age at First Marriage.* World Fertility Survey Comparative Studies No. 7. Voorburg, Netherlands: International Statistical Institute.
Smith, Peter C., M. Shahidullah, and A.N. Alacantara
    1983   *Cohort Nuptiality in Asia and the Pacific: An Analysis of WFS Surveys.* World Fertility Survey Comparative Studies No. 22. Voorburg, Netherlands: International Statistical Institute.
Spring, S.B., and J. Gruber
    1985   Relationship of DNA viruses and cervical carcinoma. *Journal of the National Cancer Institute* 75(3):589-590.
Stadel, B.
    1986   Oral contraceptives and the occurrence of disease: Clinical overview. Pp. 3-41 in A.T. Gregoire and R.G. Blye (eds.), *Contraceptive Steroids: Pharmacology and Safety.* New York: Plenum Press.
Stadel, Bruce, S. Lai, J.J. Schlesselman, and P. Murray
    1988   Oral contraceptives and premenopausal breast cancer in nulliparous women. *Contraception* 38(3):287-299.
Stone, K.M., D.A. Grimes, and L.S. Magder
    1986   Personal protection against sexually transmitted diseases. *American Journal of Obstetrics and Gynecology* 155(1):180-188.
Strobino, D.M.
    1987   The health and medical consequences of adolescent sexuality and pregnancy: A review of the literature. Pp. 93-122 in Sandra L. Hofferth and Cheryl D. Hayes (eds), *Risking the Future: Adolescent Sexuality, Pregnancy, and Childbearing*, Vol. 2. Washington, D.C.: National Academy Press.
Swan, S.H., and D.B. Petitti
    1982   A review of problems of bias and confounding in epidemiologic studies of cervical neoplasia and oral contraceptive use. *American Journal of Epidemiology* 115(1):10-18.
Swenson, I., A.R. Khan, and F.A. Jahan
    1980   A randomized, single blind comparative trial of norethindrone enanthate and depot-medroxyprogesterone acetate in Bangladesh. *Contraception* 21(3):207-215.
Tietze, Christopher
    1983   *Induced Abortion: A World Review*, 5th ed. New York: The Population Council.
Trussell, J.
    1988   Does family planning reduce infant mortality? An exchange. *Population and Development Review* 14(1):171-178.
Trussell, J., and K. Kost
    1987   Contraceptive failure in the United States: A critical review of the literature. *Studies in Family Planning* 18(5):237-283.
Trussell, J., and A.R. Pebley
    1984   The potential impact of changes in fertility on infant, child, and maternal mortality. *Studies in Family Planning* 15(6):267-280.
Trussell, J., and K.I. Reinis
    1989   Age at first marriage and age at first birth. *Population Bulletin.* ST/ESA/Series N/26. New York: United Nations.
Trussell, J., and G. Rodriguez
    1989   Heterogeneity in Demographic Research. Paper prepared for the Conference on Convergent Questions in Genetics and Demography. University of Michigan, Ann Arbor.
Turner, C.F., H.G. Miller, and L.E. Moses (eds.)
    1989   *AIDS, Sexual Behavior, and Intravenous Drug Use.* Committee on AIDS Research and the Behavioral, Social, and Statistical Sciences. Commission on Behavioral and Social Sciences and Education, National Research Council. Washington, D.C.: National Academy Press.

United Nations
  1988a Levels and Trends of Contraceptive Use as Assessed in 1987. U.N. Population Division, New York.
  1988b *Mortality of Children Under Age 5: World Estimates and Projections, 1950-2025.* Population Studies No. 105. New York: United Nations, Department of International Economic and Social Affairs.
  1988c World Demographic Estimates and Projections, 1950-2025. Department of International Economic and Social Affairs, United Nations, New York.
  1989 *Levels and Trends of Contraceptive Use as Assessed in 1988.* Publication no. ST-ESA-SER.A-110. New York: United Nations.
Vessey, M.P.
  1980 Female hormones and vascular disease: An epidemiological overview. *British Journal of Family Planning* 6(Suppl. 3):1-12.
Vessey, M.P., M. Lawless, K. McPherson, and D. Yeates
  1983 Neoplasia of the cervix uteri and contraception: A possible adverse effect of the pill. *The Lancet* 2:930-934.
Vessey, M.P., M.A. Metcalfe, K. McPherson, and D. Yeates
  1987 Urinary tract infection in relation to diaphragm use and obesity. *International Journal of Epidemiology* 16(3):441-444.
Walker, A.M., H. Jick, J.R. Hunter, A. Danford, R.N. Watkins, L. Ahadeff, and K.J. Rothman
  1981 Vasectomy and nonfatal myocardial infarction. *The Lancet* 1:13-15.
Walker, G.J., D.E. Ashley, A. McCaw, and G.W. Bernard
  1985 Maternal mortality in Jamaica: A confidential inquiry into all maternal deaths in Jamaica 1981-1983. WHO FHE/PMM/85.9.10. WHO Interregional Meeting on Prevention of Maternal Mortality, Geneva, 11-15 November.
Washington, A.E., S. Gove, J. Schachter, and R.L. Sweet
  1985 Oral contraceptives, chlamydia trachomatis infection, and inflammatory disease: A word of caution about protection. *The Journal of the American Medical Association* 253(15):2246-2250.
Weinbreck, P., V. Loustaud, F. Denis, B. Vidal, M. Mounier, and L. DeLumley
  1988 Postnatal transmission of HIV infection. *The Lancet* 1:482.
Weller, R.H., I.W. Eberstein, and M. Bailey
  1987 Pregnancy wantedness and maternal behavior during pregnancy. *Demography* 24(3):407-412.
Wilson, J.G., and R.L. Brent
  1981 Are female sex hormones teratogenic? *American Journal of Obstetrics and Gynecology* 141(5):567-580.
Wingrave, S.J., and C.R. Kay
  1982 Oral contraceptives and gallbladder disease. Royal College of General Practitioners' Oral Contraception Study. *The Lancet* 2:957-959.
Winikoff, B.
  1983 The effects of birthspacing on child and maternal health. *Studies in Family Planning* 14(10):231-245.
Winikoff, B., and M. Sullivan
  1987 Assessing the role of family planning in reducing maternal mortality. *Studies in Family Planning* 18(3):128-143.
Wolfers, David, and Susan Scrimshaw
  1975 Child survival and intervals between pregnancies in Guayaquil, Ecuador. *Population Studies* 29(3):479-496.
Wongboonsin, Kua, and John Knodel
  1988 Birth Interval and Birth Order Distributions Over Thailand's Fertility Transition. Paper presented at the National Seminar on Population, the Thai Population Association, November 10-11.
World Health Organization (Task Force on Long-acting Systemic Agents for the Regulation of Fertility)
  1978 Multinational comparative clinical evaluation of two long-acting injectable contraceptive steroids: Norethisterone oenanthate and medroxyprogesterone acetate. 2. Bleeding patterns and side effects. *Contraception* 17(5):395-406.

World Health Organization
    1981   The effect of female sex hormones on fetal development and infant health. *World Health Organization Technical Report Series* No. 657.
World Health Organization (Collaborative Study of Neoplasia and Steroid Contraceptives)
    1985a   Invasive cervical cancer and combined oral contraceptives. *British Medical Journal* 290:961-965.
World Health Organization (Secretariat)
    1985b   Measuring maternal mortality. WHO FHE/PMM/85.6.2. Interregional Meeting on Prevention of Maternal Mortality, Geneva, 11-15 November.
World Health Organization
    1986a   Depot-medroxyprogesterone acetate (DMPA) and cancer: Memorandum from a WHO Meeting. *Bulletin of the World Health Organization* 64(3):375-382.
World Health Organization (Task Force on Long-acting Systemic Agents for Fertility Regulation)
    1986b   Metabolic side-effects of injectable depot-medroxyprogesterone acetate, 150 mg three-monthly, in undernourished lactating women. *Bulletin of the World Health Organization* 64(4):587-594.
World Health Organization
    1987a   The hypertensive disorders of pregnancy. *WHO Technical Report* Series, No. 758.
World Health Organization (Task Force on Long-acting Systemic Agents for Fertility Regulation)
    1987b   A multicentered phase III comparative clinical trial of depot-medroxyprogesterone acetate given three-monthly at doses of 100 mg or 150 mg: II. The comparison of bleeding patterns. *Contraception* 35(6):591-610.
World Health Organization (International Collaborative Study of Hypertensive Disorders of Pregnancy)
    1988   Geographic variation in the incidence of hypertension in pregnancy. *American Journal of Obstetrics and Gynecology* 158(1):80-83.
Wright, N.H., M.P. Vessey, B. Kenward, K. McPherson, and R. Doll
    1978   Neoplasia and dysplasia of the cervix uteri and contraception: A possible protective effect of the diaphragm. *British Journal of Cancer* 38(2):273-279.
Zimicki, Susan
    1989   The relationship between maternal mortality and fertility. In A.M. Parnell (ed.), *Contraceptive Use and Controlled Fertility: Health Issues for Women and Children.* Washington, D.C.: National Academy Press.

Appendix
Background Papers

Reproductive Behavior and Child Survival Among Nineteenth-Century
Mormons
  Lee L. Bean, Geraldine P. Mineau, and Douglas L. Anderton

Psychosocial Consequences to Women of Contraceptive Use and Controlled
Fertility
  Ruth Dixon-Mueller

Family Planning Services Based on Reproductive Risk: A New Strategy of the
Mexican Social Security Institute
  James N. Gribble and Aurora Rabago

Mechanisms for the Association of Maternal Age, Parity, and Birth Spacing
With Infant Health
  John G. Haaga

Health Effects of Contraception
  Nancy C. Lee, Herbert B. Peterson, and Susan Y. Chu

Maternal Mortality in the European Past
  Katherine A. Lynch

On the Relationship Between Contraceptive Use and Access to Health Care in Developing Countries
   Joseph E. Potter

Abortion and Contraception
   Susan M. Rogers

Birth Interval and Birth Order Distributions Over Thailand's Fertility Transition
   Kua Wongboonsin and John Knodel

The Relationship Between Maternal Mortality and Fertility
   Susan Zimicki

Glossary

Abortion rate: The estimated number of abortions per 1,000 women ages 15-44 in a given year.

Abortion ratio: The estimated number of abortions per 1,000 live births in a given year.

Abruptio placenta: Premature detachment of the placenta from the uterus prior to delivery, which if untreated leads to fetal death, hemorrhage, and blood clotting.

Age-specific fertility rates: The number of live births occurring during a specified period per 1,000 women within a specific age group.

Amenorrhea: Absences of menses, see lactational amenorrhea.

Birth interval: The length of time between one birth outcome and the next birth outcome.

Birth order: The ordinal number of a given live birth in relation to all previous live births of the same woman (e.g., 5 is the birth order of the 5th live birth occurring to the same woman).

Child mortality rate: The annual number of deaths of children ages 1 to 5 per 1,000 live births.

Childbearing years: The reproductive age span of women, usually assumed to be from ages 15 to 44 or 49.

115

Children ever born: The total number of live births although stillbirths are sometimes included.

Cohort: A group of individuals sharing some common event or characteristic, for example, a birth cohort is a group of individuals born in the same time period.

Crude birth rate: The annual number of live births per 1,000 people in the population at midyear.

Crude death rate: The annual number of deaths per 1,000 people in the population at midyear.

Eclampsia: See pregnancy-induced hypertension.

Ectopic pregnancy: Development of the fertilized ovum outside the uterine cavity.

Endometrium: The mucous membrane lining the uterus.

Fecundity: The biological capacity to reproduce.

General fertility rate: The number of live births per 1,000 women of reproductive age (ages 15-44 and 15-49) in a given year.

Gravidity: The number or previous pregnancies a woman has had.

Gynecological age: The stage of physical or biological maturation that a girl has achieved.

Hemorrhage: Heavy or uncontrolled bleeding. As a pregnancy complication, this condition is most commonly associated with births to mothers with high parity.

Infant mortality rate: The number of deaths of infants under age 1 per 1,000 live births in a given year.

Intrapartum: Occurring during childbirth or during delivery.

Intrauterine growth retardation: Poor growth of a fetus in the uterus, resulting in low birthweight.

Lactational amenorrhea: Absence of menses following birth and associated with breastfeeding.

Laparotomy: Surgical incision through the abdominal section.

Life expectancy: The average number of remaining years of life if current levels of mortality were to continue.

Low birthweight: The condition of infants weighing less than 2,500 grams at birth.

Maternal depletion: A condition in which the mother's nutritional stores are exhausted.

Maternal mortality rate: The number of deaths of women of reproductive age in a given year per 10,000 or 100,000 women ages 15-44 (or 15-49).

Maternal mortality ratio: The number of deaths of women of reproductive age per 100,000 live births in a given year.

Natural fertility: Fertility in the absence of deliberate birth control.

Neonatal period: The first 28 days of life.

Nulliparous: Having never given birth to a viable infant.

Obstructed labor: A condition in which progress toward delivery is obstructed by an abnormality of the pelvis, by an unusually large fetal head or some other abnormal fetal presentation.

Parity: The number of previous live births a woman has had.

Pelvic inflammatory disease (PID): Ascending infection from the vaginal or cervix to the uterus, fallopian tubes, and broad ligaments.

Perinatal mortality: The combination of fetal deaths occurring after 28 weeks of gestation and infant deaths occurring at less than 1 week of life.

Placenta previa: A placenta that develops in the lower uterus so that it covers or adjoins the cervical opening of the uterus, resulting in massive, fatal hemorrhage at the time of delivery unless a cesarian section is performed.

Postneonatal period: The time between the end of the first month of life and the first birthday.

Pregnancy-induced hypertension: A condition that includes abnormally high blood pressure during pregnancy together with edema and protein in the urine, leading in the most severe cases to convulsions and death. In those cases with convulsions, the condition is called eclampsia.

Pregnancy interval: The time between pregnancies.

Primigravida: A woman pregnant for the first time.

Primiparity: The condition or fact of being primiparous.

Primiparous: Bearing or having borne one child.

Relative risk: The probability of an event occurring among those with a particular characteristic relative to the probability of the same event occurring among those without that characteristic.

Reproductive mortality: Mortality associated with pregnancy and childbirth.

Retrospective data: Information that is collected from respondents who report recalled experiences from a previous date or particular age.

Total fertility rate: The mean number of live births to a woman or to a cohort of 1,000 women of reproductive age subject to the age-specific fertility rates of a given year. The total fertility rate is a hypothetical measure, since age-specific fertility rates change from year to year.

Unobserved heterogeneity: The exclusion of relevant explanatory variables from a statistical model because they are not available to the analyst (either unobserved or unobservable).